SOCIAL SUPPORT, HEALTH, AND ILLNESS:
A COMPLICATED RELATIONSHIP

RANJAN ROY

Social Support, Health, and Illness

A Complicated Relationship

UNIVERSITY OF TORONTO PRESS
Toronto Buffalo London

ISBN 978-1-4426-4035-1

♾

Printed on acid-free, 100% post-consumer recycled paper with vegetable-based inks.

Library and Archives Canada Cataloguing in Publication

Roy, Ranjan
Social support, health, and illness : a complicated relationship /
Ranjan Roy.

Includes bibliographical references and index.
ISBN 978-1-4426-4035-1

1. Social networks – Health aspects.   2. Social networks – Therapeutic
use.   3. Patients – Social networks.   4. Chronically ill – Care.   I. Title.

RA418.R69 2011   306.461   C2011-901199-9

University of Toronto Press acknowledges the financial assistance to its
publishing program of the Canada Council for the Arts and the Ontario
Arts Council.

 Canada Council   Conseil des Arts
for the Arts   du Canada   **ONTARIO ARTS COUNCIL**
CONSEIL DES ARTS DE L'ONTARIO

University of Toronto Press acknowledges the financial support of the
Government of Canada through the Canada Book Fund for its publishing
activities.

For Allan McFarlane, MD
Professor Emeritus, Department of Psychiatry, McMaster University

Contents

Preface

This book has been in the making a very long time. My friend Dr Allan McFarlane of McMaster University (to whom this book is dedicated) invited me, a complete novice in research, to join his team of researchers investigating the relationship between life-events and morbidity and the buffers that protected individuals from succumbing to the negative effects of life-events. One buffer we investigated was social support. This was in the late 1970s and early 1980s. Since that time there has been an explosion of research in social support in all its complexities. While over the years I have written and taught on the subject, I have felt for some time that social support deserved a book (although there are numerous ones on this topic) that had a clear clinical function and explored pros and cons of social support in the clinical context.

To that end, this book is an endeavour to bring together in a single volume a synthesis of research in social support and its role in mitigating disease. But not only that. Social support can exact a heavy cost for the providers of support, such as with the caregivers of a person with Alzheimer's disease. Too much social support, such as solicitous behaviour, can be counterproductive. In other words, why and how does social support act as a buffer against the full ravages of a disease or hasten recovery and at the same time give rise to other problems.

The early research on support and health dates back to the 1970s, when Holmes and Rahe (1967) proposed that confronted with recent events individuals often succumb to morbidity. However, there were many mitigating factors or buffers which seemed to protect individuals from getting sick. Our own research, along with that of others, built on the pioneering work of Holmes and Rahe, first by refining the concept of life-events itself and incorporating social support, among other things, to examine the power of mediating factors (McFarlane, Norman, Streiner, & Roy, 1984). First, recent negative events, combined with the key factor of individual perception of an event, proved to be a better measure of a person's vulnerability to morbidity. As for social support, the intimacy factor emerged as a more powerful predictor for the strength of the buffering effect than the number of individuals in a person's social network. Since those early days, research literature has virtually exploded and many new insights have emerged.

This book is a comprehensive review of the contemporary literature, and it explores a variety of chronic disorders ranging from chronic pediatric conditions to dementia. In that process, our goal will be to highlight the complexities that are disease-specific. One of the key areas of exploration is family support and the emotional and physical cost associated with that. The cost of caregiving can be enormous. This particular problem is well researched in relation to Alzheimer's and other organic brain disorders. This is one of our key areas of investigation.

Chapter 1 is historical as well theoretical. It traces the development of the concept of social support in relation to health with emphasis on new insights. The theoretical part will explore the mechanisms that underlie social support as a buffer against morbidity. Chapters 2–8 focus on specific chronic conditions and the current state of research. Issues specific to the conditions will be highlighted, as will some of the negative consequences. Not all social support is conducive to health. Exploration of this phenomenon will be an important aspect of this book. Chapter 9 will investigate the application and efficacy of social support interventions with medically ill patients. The final chapter, apart from summarizing key findings, will explore future directions in research. The clinical significance of social support in patient care will be emphasized throughout this volume.

It is our hope that this book will have wide appeal for researchers and clinicians alike as it brings together the current state of knowledge, with all its wrinkles. For researchers, this could serve as a good source of reference, and for clinicians as a guide to take into account this critical aspects of their patients' lives.

I have many people to thank for this book. Principal among them are Allan McFarlane, Geoff Norman, and David Streiner (all of whom were at McMaster University), who put up with my shortcomings and went to extraordinary lengths to teach me the finer point of conducting a significant research undertaking. This book would not have been written but for the encouragement I received from my friend Dr Robert

Chernomas, who, upon learning that I was planning to stop writing, asked me if I was planning to be brain-dead. My wife Margaret was as usual my main source of support. I cannot thank my editor, Virgil Duff of the University of Toronto Press, enough. He has supported me in numerous ways over almost the past two decades. The same goes for Anne Laughlin, managing editor of the University of Toronto Press. This book is dedicated to Allan McFarlane, MD, Professor Emeritus, Department of Psychiatry, McMaster University.

REFERENCES

Holmes, T., & Rahe, R. (1967). The social readjustment scale. *J. Psychosomatic Research, 11*, 213–218.

McFarlane, A., Norman, G., Streiner, D., & Roy, R. (1984). Characteristics and correlates of effective and ineffective social support. *J. Psychosomatic Research, 28*, 501–510.

SOCIAL SUPPORT, HEALTH, AND ILLNESS:
A COMPLICATED RELATIONSHIP

1 Social Support and Health: An Overview

Young and Willmott (1957), in their classic study of an east London community in the late 1950s, described the characteristics of a close-knit, homogeneous community with an intricate web of relationships between family members and the extended family. It is a story of mutual obligations characterized by love and affection and strong family bonds. Mothers, in general, could rely on their married daughters to remain a part of the family and provide help when necessary. These daughters also brought their husbands into their orbit and thus became part of the extended family. Sons, by contrast, were more inclined to become a part of their in-laws' extended family system. The fact that these kinships were so prevalent in an urban setting was a source of considerable surprise. Young and Willmott wrote of the residents of Bethnal Green (the community they investigated), faced with relocation, 'that very few people wish to leave the east end. They are attached to Mum and Dad, to the markets, to the pubs and settlements, to Club Row and the London Hospital' (p. 186).

In today's terms, this east London community would fall into the category of a cohesive neighbourhood with strong family and social ties. Young and Willmott reported on the people who chose to be relocated. One stark finding was that the family and social ties were considerably loosened in the process. The flavour of Young and Willmott's Bethnal Green of the 1950s can only be savoured in long-running English soaps such as *Coronation Street*. One very obvious change in the East End of London is its multicultural mix, dominated to a measurable extent by Bangladeshis.

Roy (2006) recently noted the array and types of families that were virtually unknown when Young and Willmott wrote their seminal

book. Not only has the nuclear family descended into a minority position in North America, the overall family picture has been enormously
complicated by single parents, a high divorce rate, in-vitro fertilization,
gay relationships with the right to adopt children, and complicated
family relationships brought on by blended and other forms of families. And yet, family remains the most important source of support. In
urban middle-class families, it is not at all unusual for children to live
far away from their parents. In an aging society, these developments
have far-reaching consequences. The 'burden' of care for an elderly
unwell person often falls on an elderly partner who may also have
significant health problems. In short, the very notion of family carries
diverse meanings. At the same time, at a fundamental level, family still
serves the same function, from raising children to providing mutual
support, and arguably remains the most important source of support
for its members. All these issues will be explored in depth throughout
this volume. This chapter is divided into three sections, examining: (1)
the work of Caplan and Cobb, the early protagonists of social support;
(2) research during the 1980s on the buffering role of social support;
and (3) the mechanisms underlying the buffering or mediating aspects
of social support.

Caplan, Cobb, and Others: The Early Protagonists

A common saying in the English-speaking world is that 'a problem
shared is a problem halved.' This simple, common-sense observation
highlights the role that our friends and family members play in helping us cope with the vicissitudes, big and small, that we encounter in
our daily lives. Two early protagonists of social support, Gerald Caplan
(1974) and Sidney Cobb (1976), contributed much in promoting systematic investigation of the role of social support in mitigating morbidity, and they are worthy of our attention. Cobb, in particular, has an
impressive record of investigation on various aspects of social support.
   Gerald Caplan (1974), in his seminal book 'Support System and Community Mental Health,' noted that the 'best known and most ubiquitous support system in all societies is the marital and family group.
Most cultures develop definite rules that legislate the reciprocal obligations that bind the kinsfolk together' (p. 8). He goes on to note that
in contemporary urban societies the slow and not so slow decline of
family support has been supplanted, to some degree, by voluntary and
government institutions. This decline of family support has profound

and complex consequences for the availability of social support for our ever-aging population.

Caplan cast a very wide net to explore the support network, including the role of the nurse in maternal and child care and that of the schools in shaping healthy children. He identified three critical functions of social support: (1) Social aggregates provide persons with a sense of self-worth through validation and may act as a buffer against disease; (2) A support system may act as a refuge or sanctuary to which a person might return for rest and recuperation; and (3) A 'support system implies an enduring pattern of continuous or intermittent ties that play a significant part in maintaining the psychological and physical integrity of the individual over time' (1974, p. 7).

Caplan's vision was to prevent mental illness in the community through the promotion of public health programs. One critical, if not the central, element of his plan was to develop a cohesive community in which support and help was available to an individual from multiple sources, which he termed the 'support system.' As our subsequent journey through this volume will show, Caplan's recognition of the central role of family as the primary source of support in the mitigation of morbidity is borne out by research.

Sidney Cobb (1976) classified social support as: (1) information leading the subject to believe that he is cared for and loved; (2) information leading the subject to believe he is esteemed and valued; and (3) information leading the subject to believe that he belongs to a network of communication and mutual obligation. His paper provides empirical evidence to support the power of social support under diverse circumstances. His intention in providing this evidence is to explore the mechanisms underlying social support that facilitate coping with crisis and adaptation to change.

Cobb reported on the role of social support in pregnancy-related complications, citing the work of Nuckolls et al. (1972), whose study showed the power of social support in cushioning women from such complications. Women confronted with a high frequency of life-changes had no increase in complications, "presumably because of some protective effect exerted by high level of social support" (p. 302). In relation to hospitalization, Cobb concluded that the evidence showed that treating patients with myocardial infarcts (heart attacks) at home as opposed to a hospital carried no greater risk of death. The mechanism by which staying at home proved equally beneficial seemed to be associated with the supportive environment of the home. (However, with advancing knowledge about cardiac care, it is no longer advisable to try and treat a heart attack patient at home.)

In his exhaustive review of the beneficial effects of social support, Cobb discussed such wide-ranging situations as employment termination, retirement, and the threat of death. His conclusion was firm and unequivocal: 'We have seen strong and quite often hard evidence, repeated over a variety of transitions in the life cycle from birth to death, that social support is protective" (p. 310). Cobb and his colleagues wrote extensively on social support research, as the following sample demonstrates.

Cancer has a way of pushing people away from patients and diminishing their sources of support. This was theme of a paper by Cobb and Erbe (1978). The loss of significant roles is common in seriously ill cancer patients, which has a direct impact on the network of relationship associated with those roles. The network subsides. Reduced participation in social activities occurs at a time when 'support networks are being demoralized by the "what do you say to a-cancer-patient syndrome"' This proposition was supported by what Roy (2007) described as a ever-shrinking support system that he observed among chronic pain sufferers.

In this thoughtful essay, Cobb and Erbe make a number of suggestions to increase the circle of support. First and foremost, counselling has to be an essential part of overall treatment. Among other tasks, the counsellor must see the family and friends, and not just the patient, as her primary responsibility. Equally important is the need to identify and make a distinction between effective and ineffective support systems. People tend to shy away from a terminally ill patient at a time when the need for, indeed the value of, social support is perhaps most critical. Cobb (1976) cites a study that revealed a clear relationship between the risk of poor health due to bereavement and that due to low social support. However, when these widows received intervention to promote social support, health improved for most of them.

Kasl, Gore, and Cobb (1975) investigated the experience of job loss and its consequences on health symptoms and health behaviour. Social support was investigated to assess its buffering effect in two settings – rural and urban. The findings were tentative at best. The authors noted that 'if we accept the proposition that in the rural setting, the social community and the social support system are less affected by the plant closing than in the urban setting, then we, at least, make the observation that a strong social support system may act as if to moderate and reduce the influence of other variables, whether they be characteristics of the person or the objective experience' (p. 119). In short, the strength and availability of social support had only a nominal effect, even in a rural setting.

While the latter study's findings pointed, albeit modestly, in the right direction, the review of Caplan, Cobb, & French (1975) found a negative association between the cessation of smoking and social support). Based on several studies, the conclusion reached was that for people who smoked in socially supportive situations more as a social habit rather than to relieve tension, and whose smoking was reinforced by group norms, social support for smoking played a complex role. The authors concluded that social support and job stress interacted such that decreases in distress coincided with decreases in the quit rate only for persons with low social support. In the absence of hard evidence, the explanation for the finding, counter to common sense, was that when social support is high, the level of job stress may be less of a motivating factor in the cessation of smoking. The authors urged more research to explore these tentative observations. The very notion that social support could serve a negative function is now supported by much research evidence in relation to a certain type of spousal support (see chapter 3). However, the critical message of the above review is that socially sanctioned behaviour, however harmful, seems immune to the buffering role of social support. On the contrary, social support may indeed reinforce the harmful activity, whatever that may be.

The final paper we present in this section is only indirectly related to social support. Chen and Cobb (1960), in one of their earlier papers, presented a comprehensive review of the literature on family structure and its impact on health and disease. The idea that people in marriage or partnership relationship enjoyed better health than single persons was reported by Chen and Cobb, and they cited a number of studies, the earliest ones dating back to 1940s (Ciocco, 1940, 1941). This observation has been supported by a huge body of research in subsequent years (Roy, 2006).

Summary

Our goal in this introductory section is simply to trace the emergence of social support as having a significant role in heath and illness. The work of Young and Willmott gives us a glimpse of a lost world which may still exist in small towns and villages, but has largely disappeared

from large urban centres. The nuclear family is now a minority phenomenon. Yet, our brief review of the early work of Caplan and Cobb
reveals the complexities that surround the concept of social support. It
is not universally positive. The very concept of social support has been
applied in wide-ranging problems as redundancy and the cessation of
smoking.

Several themes emerge from this brief incursion into the past:

1   The central role of the family in mitigating morbidity.
2   The value of social intervention programs to promote social support.
3   The value of social support in widely divergent situations and set-
    tings.
4   The negative fallout from social support.
5   A relationship between marriage and health.

All these issues will emerge and re-emerge in subsequent chapters.
These early protagonists made observations based on clinical and
sometimes empirical evidence. Much of these early observations have
been affirmed by empirical evidence. In the section that follows, we
discuss the buffering or mediating role of social support in different
situations in more recent times, mainly the 1980s, during which there
was an explosion of research in this area.

The Buffering Role of Support: Research during the 1980s

The decade of the 1980s witnessed a veritable explosion of social support research. One area that attracted huge attention was the buffering
or mediating role of social support to mitigate, moderate, or eliminate
the negative consequences of stress and morbidity. The capacity of
social support to protect human beings from the noxious consequences of negative events lies at the very heart of social support research.
Without this particular role, social support as a topic of research could
never have attained its prominence. We survey the research scene by
first presenting a brief summary of the review papers on the topic; second, we discuss a selected sample of the buffering literature, primarily
to highlight its relevance with very divergent populations with equally
diverse problems. We begin by presenting an overview that examines
four major review papers that appeared during the 1980s on the buffering function.

Review of Reviews

Thoits (1982) reviewed the literature of the previous twenty years, and noted that several issues remained problematic with the buffering hypothesis. Among those Thoits identified was inadequate conceptualization of the very concept of social support. Her second concern was that many studies failed to take into account the changing nature of support. Life-changes could alter the number of individuals in the support system.

Based on this extensive review Thoits concluded that the buffering role of social support should be interpreted with extreme caution because of inadequate conceptualization and the fact that the direct and interactive effects of life-change and social support may have been inadvertently confounded in cross-sectional studies. She made the important observation that life-events were capable of altering the support available, and support may indeed lower the risk of encountering life-events. The final concern noted in this review was that the theoretical relationships between life-events, social support and, psychological disturbance were not adequately clarified.

Wallston and colleagues (1983) conducted a review of the relevant literature in terms of (1) onset of illness; (2) utilization of health services; (3) adherence to medical regimen; and (4) recovery, rehabilitation, and adaptation to illness. They were cognizant, as the previous author was, of the broadness of the concept of social support, and discussed it from several perspectives. Because of the retrospective nature of social support, causal association between support and outcome was problematic. A related problem was the use of a wide array of instruments to measure social support, which made comparison between studies very difficult.

In relation to the onset of illness, many shortcomings, discussed above, in the research methodology emerged. A number of studies failed to find any association between onset of illness and social support. Evidence to the contrary was also somewhat less than convincing. In the category of social support as a buffer against stress, responses were mixed. Prospective studies designed to test statistical interaction failed to yield consistent outcomes, thereby putting in question the universality of the buffering hypothesis. However, retrospective statistical interaction data, with some limitations, did provide relatively consistent support for the buffering hypotheses. The actual number of these studies was few. The general conclusions in the areas of utilization of health services and social support, and of recovery and rehabilitation, were not dissimilar. However, a few studies did provide support for a positive relationship between social support and stress and service utilization. Another area where progress in conceptualization was notable was the development of models to differentiate between sources of support, such as kin versus friends. Wallston and colleagues proposed improved methodology and refinement of the concept of social support. In addition, they made a strong case for a standardization of instruments to measure it.

Cohen and Wills (1985) in their comprehensive review of literature with stringent criteria for inclusion arrived at very different conclusions than the two reviews above. They drew a distinction between support as a main effect and support as a stress buffer. This paper, one of the most extensive and conceptually sound reviews, found much support both as a main effect and as a buffer. Evidence for a main-effect model was established when the support instruments deliberately measured a person's level of integration in a large network of relationships. However, while feeling integrated into a social network may enhance a sense of well-being, this did not necessarily translate into better coping with stressful situations. It was surmised that these results could be attributed either to a more general effect of the social network on feelings of stability, predictability, and self-worth. One noteworthy conclusion of this review was that while a single confidant was sufficient for stress buffering, a large network of social relationships was not.

As for the buffering model, the conclusion of Cohen and Wills was that social support provided consistent evidence for the buffering effect as long as certain conditions were met. They consisted of (1) methodological and statistical criteria, (2) the ability of the instruments measuring support to assess perceived availability of a support function, and (3) a requirement that the support functions must be those that enhanced broadly used coping abilities.

Another point of note was the assertion that the main-effect and the buffering hypotheses were not mutually exclusive. Social integration and functional support represented different processes through which social resources affect well-being. There were several other issues clarified by this review. Perception of available support systems was found to operate as a buffer. However, there was no examination of the process of drawing on a support system in the face of stressful events. Perception of available support would appear to be a sensitive indicator of buffering effects due to the fact that the buffering qualities of social support are presumed to be cognitively mediated. The effectiveness of support seemed to be effective in both acute as well as chronic situations. Quality of support also emerged as an important issue. The buffering effect of marital satisfaction is a case in point. Such effects are influenced to one degree or another by gender, social class, and type of stressor. The authors noted that the findings in relation to these variables were somewhat equivocal. This review found significant evidence in the research literature to confirm the buffering effect of social support.

Another paper arrived at very different conclusions than the previous ones. Alloway and Bebbington (1987) conducted a comprehensive review of the research literature on the buffering effect of social support in relation to minor affective disturbances. They addressed some of the problems that were noted by our previous reviewers, which ranged from problems with the operational definitions and measuring of social support to the unsatisfactory methodologies applied to analyse the buffering effect to issues with measuring events. They made a number of suggestions that would avoid the methodological pitfalls noted and produce more reliable results. The authors conclude: 'Our review leads to the conclusion that evidence for a buffering role of social support is inconsistent, reflecting methodological differences between studies but probably also indicating that buffering effects are not of dramatic proportions' (p. 91).

Summary

Only one (Cohen and Wills, 1985) out of the four reviews we examined reported, at best, the questionable power of the buffering effect. Common concerns reported by researchers of that era were definitional and methodological shortcomings that were clearly in need of refinement. There seemed to be consensus on the complexity that surrounded the very concept of social support, but at the same time there was a recognition that the buffering effect, to one degree or another, could be effective. Individuals confronted with vicissitudes of life were protected by the presence of intimates. Another area of clarification was the recognition that a personal support system was largely responsible for the buffering effect in some situations and not in others. A clear distinction between network support and individual support was delineated. In the following section we present a selection of studies that demonstrate some of these issues, and further confirm the complexity of the buffering function in divergent situations.

Divergent populations and problems and the buffering effect: A Psychinfo search with the terms 'Social Support and Health and Buffer' between 1980 and 1990 produced 136 articles. What we present here is a small, select sample. As the rest of this volume is concerned with the impact of social support for medically ill patients, we devote the rest of this chapter to examining the research literature during the 1980s for non-medical problems and populations. Our reason for this diversion is to show the breadth of the notion of buffering in situations ranging from natural disaster to urban living.

We have selected a group of research reports that broadly fall into the following categories: stress and buffering in a group of community residents (McFarlane, Norman, Streiner, & Roy, 1983; Oxley, Barrera, & Sadalla, 1981; Wilcox, 1981); job stress (LaRocco, Tetrick, & Meder, 1989; Ross, Altmaier, & Russell, 1989; Westman, Eden, & Shirom, 1985); women and wives (Parry & Shapiro, 1986; Rosen & Moghadam, 1988; Tetzloff & Barrera, 1987).

Community-Based Studies

In this section we review three studies with different and yet overlapping objectives and methodologies (McFarlane et al., 1983: Oxley et al., 1981; Wilcox, 1981). Oxley and colleagues (1981) conducted a type of study, namely, on the role the community as a buffer against stress, that has virtually disappeared from the literature. This study investigated the size of a community as a potential determinant of the availability of social support. They tested the network size and the average social support provided by network members. A telephone survey of four communities of varying sizes was conducted. One hundred and sixty residents answered questions about the social support they received from their network members. In broad terms, the size of the community had an inverse relationship to the availability of social support – the smaller the size of the community, the better average social support. Urbanization, the authors noted, had an adverse relationship to social support. One point of note about this study is that family members were deliberately excluded from it to get an accurate picture of community support. Social segmentalization, a fact of urban living, emerged as a significant mediator of this relationship. One recommendation to emerge from this study was to identify the characteristics of small towns to promote more supportive social relationships in larger communities. It is noteworthy that some of the issues noted in this study can be found in the contemporary research on 'healthy community.'

Wilcox's (1981) study, by contrast, was one of the earlier ones to measure the impact of intimate relationships in mitigating stress. A multitude of factors influence the relationship between stressful life-events and psychological 'judgment.' Wilcox designed this study to investigate one factor, namely, social support for that relationship. A community-based sample of 320 residents completed two sets of questionnaires on social support and two psychological distress scales and a stressful life-events scale. The buffering hypothesis was tested between life-events and psychological distress for each of the two support measures in predicting each of the two psychological distress variables.

All four hypothesis were supported, although quality rather than quantity of support accounted for much greater variance. However, the actual buffering effect was modest in statistical terms. The authors noted that this finding was in agreement with a much earlier study (Lowenthal and Haven, 1968), which found that the quality of a person's supportive network, mainly in the form of a single intimate relationship, rather than the quantity of support accounted for much of the buffering effect. Wilcox's study was important, as it tried to operationalize support in a 'manner that would capture some of the richness of the construct' (p. 383). Still, the author conceded that the results of this study, while finding evidence for the buffering effect, failed to explain the underlying mechanism. Having noted a dearth of research on the concept of social support, Wilcox recommended further research.

Our final study was a prospective, community-based longitudinal study with a population of 428 (McFarlane et al., 1983). The study led to refinement of a number of critical issues such as the influence of the dimensions or quality of events, specificity of the quality of event, and its impact, which was in turn controlled by perception of the event and availability of social support. As for the dimension of events, the authors' earlier work had shown that only the events that were judged by the subjects as being undesirable and the events that were uncontrollable showed a significant relationship with the measure of distress. Further refinement was incorporated in the present study by scoring stressful events in three sub-categories: all events; neutral or undesirable, no-control events; and controllable events. The Social Relationship Scale was used to derive two measures of social support, namely, the quality of helpfulness of social network and its extent.

There were some critical findings. First, there seemed to be a high level of correlation between stressful events over time, suggesting that there were consistent patterns of exposure to stressful events within a population. Second, patterns of health were found to be stable over time. Stressful events did have an impact on health status, but the correlations were significantly lower than in previously reported cross-sectional studies. Third, better health was associated with less exposure to stressful events. This meant that availability of support served a critical function in reducing exposure to stressful events. Other findings in relation to social support were that the extent or the size of the network did not exert any buffering effect. On the other hand, individuals who reported smaller, but overall more helpful networks also reported that their inner core of intimates were considerably more helpful. Most critically, a reciprocal relationship was found between social supports and stressful events.

Some of the more intriguing findings of this study were further replicated and refined in a subsequent report by McFarlane and colleagues (McFarlane, Norman, Streiner, & Roy, 1984), which indicated that subjects who reported least helpful social support also experienced significantly more stressful life-events in the previous five years also reported having large social network. One notable finding was that subjects with a smaller network not only experienced less stressful events, but derived support primarily from spouse and close family relationship – an observation reported by many previous investigators.

Summary

These three studies revealed certain trends in research. Apart from improved methodology, there also was a shift away from the notion of network support to a more precise definition of the sources of support. Number was less important than quality. McFarlane's study was significant because it demonstrated the power of the intimates within a network to provide stability of health over time, experience less negative events, and serve a preventive function. The role of the intimates rather than network support emerged as a vital finding with clinical implications. An altogether higher level of sophistication was notable in the effort to classify quality of events in terms of their desirability, controllability, and predictability. The buffering hypothesis was supported in the McFarlane study and affirmed the power of buffering to prevent stressful life-events when support was provided by intimates.

Stress of Work and Social Support

We report here on three very different studies concerned with the role of social support in work situations: LaRocco, Tetrick, and Meder (1989); Ross, Altmaier, & Russell (1989); and Westman, Eden, & Shirom (1985).

Westman and associates (1985) investigated the impact of social support in a Israeli population of male smokers and quitters. All subjects were 35 years of age and older. The purpose of this study was to investigate smoking intensity and job stress and the buffering effect of social support. Results were unequivocal in showing that among factors such as job intensity, hours of work, and work addiction, lack of social support was positively associated with smoking intensity.

Subjects with low peer support smoked significantly more than those with high levels of such support. Moreover, for subjects reporting low support, more job stressors were negatively related to cessation than among those reporting high support, thus confirming, according to the authors, the support-buffer hypothesis. Critically, in support of a previous study (Caplan, Cobb, & French, 1975), social support, the authors noted, could indeed be detrimental to the smoker if the attitudes and behaviours of the support system reinforced smoking. This study is noteworthy for the fact that the source of social support may vary depending on the problem and the circumstances. In this study peer support and its quality were deciding factors in the effectiveness of the buffering hypothesis.

The next study (LaRocco, Tetrick, & Meder, 1989) is of a totally different order. Stress and well-being were tested in a group of military physicians (n=86), dentists (n=40), and nurses (n=94). As in the previous study, job characteristics, job stress, attitudes and social support, and health outcome was investigated. Sources of social support were supervisors, peers, subordinates, and significant others, which included spouses and parents. Results were mixed and somewhat counterintuitive. Dentists reported greater social support and satisfaction than nurses. Hence, their report of more health worries and report of more negative health outcomes was unexpected and somewhat inexplicable.

Nurses reported more control and influence over decisions than either the dentists or physicians. And yet, they perceived more responsibility for others and more uncertainty or lack of predictability of events than either the physicians or the dentists. They were the least satisfied as a group.

Physicians reported the highest professional orientation, the lowest administrative orientation, but lower satisfaction with the organization. With the exception of support from significant others, support from other sources, while statistically significant, was weak. Occupational groups varied in their perception of social support from peers and significant others. However, dentists reported the most support and nurses the least. The confounding fact was that social support alone could not explain a higher level of negative outcomes, especially among the dentists, who also reported having greater social support. The authors proposed that there might be a direct link between environmental stressors and health outcome, especially psychological well-being.

Our final study in this section reports an investigation of work-related stress and social support in 169 doctoral-level counsellors recruited nationwide (Ross, Altmaier, & Russell, 1989). Questionnaires were mailed to 257 subjects, and 169 responded. Subjects were asked if they had experienced a stressful life-event and to rate the stressfulness of the event on a seven-point scale. Social support elicited two types of support: (1) supervisors, co-workers, spouse, and friends/relatives; (2) those that elicited relational provisions such as attachment that provided the individual with a sense of safety and security, a sharing common interests, and reassurance of worth.

The results were complex. Events rated as the most stressful included clients committing suicide, counsellors being physically threatened, and clients threatening homicide. Counsellor and setting variables accounted for 15% of the variance in the number of stressful events reported. The social support measures explained only 3.5 to 11.4% of the variance of the burnout scores. Supervisor support was significantly related to the burnout phenomenon. Counsellors with a high level of support from supervisors also reported lower levels of stress and higher levels of personal accomplishment.

There are several point of note. Work-related stresses were clearly identified and the fact that they had the potential of causing burnout. Of all the supports available to the counsellors, one that held sway was supervisor support. Curiously, married counsellors reported more stressful events than their single counterparts. Minority counsellors were also susceptible to more stressors. In the work situation, the availability of more than adequate supervisor support is a prerequisite to a healthy work environment.

Summary

Peer support, supervisory support, and somewhat ineffectual intimate support would describe the main features of the three studies. Peer support is also not without qualification, as we witnessed in the cessation of smoking study. In the study of military personnel, intimate support failed to produce a buffering effect. In the other two studies, however, the buffering hypothesis received some confirmation.

Women, Vulnerability, and Social Support

In this section we report on three studies investigating life-events, social support, and psychiatric disorder in a community sample of 193 women (Parry and Shapiro, 1986); divorcing mothers and social support (Tetzloff & Barrera, 1987); and social support and well-being in military wives (Rosen & Moghadam, 1990).

Parry and Shapiro (1986) engaged in a study of psychological vulnerability in a group of working-class women to test the stress-buffering hypothesis vis-à-vis independent effects. The sample consisted of 193 working-class women selected from a larger sample of 812 subjects. In addition to measuring life-events, three types of supportive measures were included: instrumental social support, expressive social support, and intimacy. Psychiatric morbidity was measured using standardized instruments including the Beck Depression Inventory.

The authors found support for both theoretical positions. They found that 33% of the unsupported and 10% of supported cases had suffered a severe event, but only 10% of supported and 5% of the unsupported women were without such an event. They noted that 'there was a consistent finding of a significant association between both forms of social support (expressive and instrumental) and psychological well-being, although in a cross sectional study it is not possible to infer the direction of cause, particularly between social support deficits and depression' (p. 322). Findings supported the view that life-event threat and social support each have a significant, but modest independent effect on psychological distress. While the authors disagreed with the prevailing view that a stress-buffering model was theoretically more interesting or had more clinical significance than an independent-effects model, they did agree that individuals who had suffered a major life-event and who lacked social support were at greater risk for psychiatric morbidity than their socially supported counterparts.

Our next study investigated the effects on general well-being of perceived social support, stress, and the stress–support interaction in a group of military wives (Rosen & Moghadam, 1988). Much of military wives' stress was due to the absence of their partners. Letters were mailed to 3000 women married to soldiers. A total of 947 subjects returned completed questionnaires. Measures included a general well-being questionnaire, and a social-support questionnaire that included four questions: (1) Are you friendly with another military wife in your husband's unit? (2) How often do you talk with another military wife from your husband's unit? (3) How often do you and your husband get together with couples from his unit? and (4) Can you count on another military wife in your husband's unit for help with a personal or family problem? As for the measurement of stress, the focus was on the ongoing strains common to all military wives rather than on occurrence of life-events.

First and foremost, results indicated that stress was significantly related to well-being only for the group that did not have support. Major predictors of social support included husband's rank, type of unit, and stress. Higher levels of stress predicted higher levels of social support. Authors attributed this to their observation that stress stimulated adaptation in most individuals. The buffering effect was evident in the behaviour of the wives with healthy coping behaviour who enlisted the support of other wives during times of stress.

Our final study in this section tested the hypothesis that there exists a match between effective social support and the needs elicited by particular stressors (Tetzloff & Barrera, 1987). It was tested using interview data from 73 women who had recently separated from their husbands. Assessment instruments included questionnaires on stress related to divorce, supportive functions, perceived availability of social support, psychological distress, and depressive symptoms.

Results did not find support for the hypothesis. The authors speculated that one reason for this discrepant finding was the vary specialized nature of the subjects. Given that divorced mothers may typically experience high levels of parenting stress relative to the general population, low levels of stress may simply be absent in these mothers. It is indeed possible that even well-supported individuals (given the power of stressors) may show signs of psychological distress that may approximate relatively those of unsupported individuals. On the basis of the null finding, the authors recommended that an effective way to prevent various types of distress for recently separated mothers would be to ensure that they receive tangible supports. The importance of providing information on child-rearing and parenting-oriented divorce support groups was emphasized.

Summary

Our three studies involving female subjects in diverse situations produced very mixed outcomes in terms of finding support for the buffering effect. With the military wives the buffering hypothesis held when the perceived source of support was other military wives (Rosen & Moghadam, 1988). Friends and intimates did not prove to be significant sources of support for these women who were separated from their military husbands. With the divorcing mothers, results did not support the specificity of a social-support buffering effect (Tetzloff & Barrera, 1987). The study involving working-class women found evidence for the perspective that life-event threat and social support each had a significant but modest independent effect on psychological distress (Parry & Shapiro, 1986). It is noteworthy that each of these studies varied in methodologies, the nature of stressors, and even the most effective sources of support. Despite these differences, their common goal was to seek confirmation for and evidence in support of the buffering effect. The relationship between life-event-induced stress and the power of social support to protect appears to be very complex indeed.

Physiological Evidence for the Buffering Hypothesis

In this final section we present three review papers on the psycho-physiological evidence for the buffering function of social support: Geiser, 1989; Robles & Klecolt-Glaser, 2003; and Uchino, 2006. It should be noted that here we have departed from the rest of the chapter's adherence to the literature of the 1980s. Our reason is simple. This particular topic is not central to the rest of this volume, and we also attempt to give our reader some idea of the progress made over the years in our understanding of the psycho-physiological changes that accompany psychosocial stress.

Leonard Pearlin (1989), in a very thoughtful paper, made the plea that information should not be treated simply as data that need to be controlled statistically; and that researchers must examine the bearing of these data on each domain of the stress process: exposure to and the meaning of stressors, access to stress mediators, and psychological and physical, and behavioural, manifestations of stress.

Twenty years ago there existed a substantial body of research linking absence of social support to immune deficiency disorders (Geiser, 1989).

The findings, in general terms, supported the notion that decreases in measures of immune status accompanied a variety of stressful life-events. The role of social support as a mediator was also supported. Nevertheless, Geiser (1989) in his comprehensive review of the relevant literature arrived at somewhat guarded conclusions. A predominance of retrospective and cross-sectional studies raised significant methodological issues questioning the findings. The issue of mechanism was also moot. In conclusion, Geiser noted, first, that social support was a multifaceted construct influenced by a number of variables, including social support. The reports in his reviews were just the beginning of examining the influence of social support on a person's immune status. Longitudinal prospective studies and multi-modal assessment could resolve some of the problems encountered by the early researchers.

Over the years the power of an intimate (spousal or partner) relationship to buffer against negative events has gained considerable momentum, and for solid reasons, as this salient finding is backed by powerful empirical evidence. The review paper we shall presently discuss presents a very complex picture of this common-sense proposition.

Robles and Klecolt-Glaser (2003), in an in-depth review of the literature related to physiological pathways through which marital relationships influenced health, unravelled the complex nature of this relationship. First, they noted that empirical evidence provided ample evidence for the proposition that married individuals reported greater happiness and a lower risk of depression than unmarried individuals. The non-married population was also at a higher risk for a whole host of diseases. The stress/social support hypothesis was the main explanation for better health among married individuals. The key quest of this review was to explore the negative health consequences of a stressful marital relationship on individuals. The weight of the evidence suggested that marital strain was capable of compromising cardiovascular, endocrine, and immune functions. Chronic social stressors showed a strong relationship with health outcome, which included responses to infectious diseases and wound healing. The authors noted that much of this research was conducted with relatively healthy couples, which placed limitations on the generalizability of the findings.

Our final review paper poses a broad question: 'How does social support influence physical health outcome' (Uchino, 2006). The relationships between social support and cardiovascular, neuro-endocrine, and immune functions are subjected to a comprehensive review of the relevant research literature. Overall, the findings support the stress/social support buffering hypothesis. Uchino noted that research findings provided ample evidence to demonstrate a link between social support and atherosclerosis, lower blood pressure, and the progression of diagnosed cardiovascular disease. As for the neuro-endocrine function, there was a dearth of studies making that link. On the other hand, some of the strongest associations have been found between social support and immune systems. Social support has been shown to predict better immune function. Ucino noted that despite these 'promising links,' there had to be more focus on social support in the context of the entire lifespan. He vary carefully plots a direction for future research.

Summary

The only meaningful observation we can make on the basis of our cursory review is that over a period of two decades or so, the intricate biological relationship between stress and heath has progressed in leaps and bounds. Even on a day-to-day basis we hear about stress and heart disease or how a myocardial infarct (heart attack) was brought on by sudden exposure to severe stressors. On the other hand, each reviewer was careful to point out the limitations of our contemporary knowledge and how much more research is required to continue to unfold the role of sole support in the mitigation of morbidity or even mortality.

Conclusion

The 1980s experienced an explosion of research on the role of social support in buffering or protecting individuals from succumbing to mental and physical disorders. The Psychinfo search between 1980 and 1989 using the term social support produced 4701 hits; 'social support and buffering' produced 560 hits. The refinements, in terms of both conceptual clarification and research methodologies, was nothing short of breathtaking. A clear move away from clustering all events as somehow having negative consequences to a refinement of events into various categories, the emergence of spousal or partner relationship as being the most powerful buffer, a need for specific social support in differing situations, and improving methodologies that vastly improve the predictability of negative events on morbidity is but a short list of the progress made during that decade.

Our modest goal in this chapter was to give the reader an overview of the progression in our understanding of social support in all its intricacies and complexities by tracking the early literature and highlighting the contribution of research during a critical decade in furthering our understanding of this concept.

This book has several limitations. The literature, in the main, is Western and almost every issue discussed in this volume has a Judeo-Christian bias. We do not know if intimate relationships have the same buffering power in other cultures. We have cited literature from other cultures, but not in a systematic way, and certainly not enough to draw any meaningful conclusions. The other limitation (and perhaps its strength) is the book's singular focus on the role of the intimate relationship in its buffering effect. In recent years, there has been an explosion of sociological literature addressing issues such as social capital, spirit level, societal justice, and so on. This volume, because of its clinical focus, did not examine that very important body of literature. Our clinical focus may also be viewed by many as somewhat limiting. Nevertheless, intimate relationships and their buffering power are at the core of this book. In the rest of this volume we turn our attention to the clinical understanding and role of social support with a variety of medical conditions.

REFERENCES

Alloway, R., & Bebbington, P. (1987). The buffer theory of social support – a review of the literature. *Psychological Medicine, 17*, 91–108.

Caplan, G. (1974). *Support systems and community mental health.* New York: Behavioral Publications.

Caplan, R., Cobb, S., & French, J. (1975). Relationships of cessation of smoking with job stress, personality, and social support. *J. Applied Psychol., 60*, 211–219.

Chen, E., & Cobb, S. (1960). Family structure in relation to health and disease: A review of the literature. *J. Chron. Dis., 12*, 544–567.

Ciocco, A. (1940). On the mortality in husbands and wives. *Human Biol., 12*, 508–513.

Ciocco, A. (1941). On the interdependence of the length of life of husband and wife. *Human Biol., 13*, 505–512.

Cobb, S. (1976). Social support as a moderator of life-stress. *Psychosomatic Medicine, 38*, 300–314.

Cobb, S., & Erbe, C. (1978). Social support for the cancer patient. *Forum on Medicine, 1*, 24–29.

Cohen, S., & Wills, T. (1985). Stress, social support, and the buffering hypothesis. *Psychological Bulletin, 98*, 310–357.

DeJong Gierveld, J., & Van Tilburg, T. (1987). The partner as source of social support in problem and non-problem situations. *J. Soc. Behav. & Personality, 2*, 191–200; *Clin. Psychol. Rev., 9*, 689–715.

Geiser, D. (1989). Psychosocial influences on human immunity. *Clinical Psychology Review, 9*: 689–715.

Kasl, S., Gore, S., & Cobb, S. (1975). The experience of losing a job: Reported changes in health, symptoms and illness behavior. *J. Psychosom. Res., 37*, 106–122.

LaRocco, J., Tetrick, L., & Meder, D. (1989). Differences in perception of work environment conditions, job attitudes, and health beliefs among military physicians, dentists, and nurses. *Military Psychology, 1*, 135–151.

Lowenthal, M., & Haven, C. (1968). Interaction and adaptation: Intimacy as a critical variable. *Am. Sociological Rev., 33*, 20–30.

McFarlane, A., Norman, G., Streiner, D., & Roy, R. (1983). The process of social stress: Stable, reciprocal, and mediating relationships. *J. Health & Social Behav. 24*, 160–173.

McFarlane, A., Norman, G., Streiner, D., & Roy, R. (1984). Characteristics and correlates of effective and ineffective social supports. *J. Psychosom. Res., 28*, 501–510.

Murphy, S. (1984). After Mount St. Helen: Disaster stress research. *J. Psychosocial Nursing and Mental Health Services, 22*, 9–18.

Nuckolls, K., Cassel, J., & Kaplan, B. (1972). Psychosocial assets, life crisis and the prognosis of pregnancy. *Am. J. Epidemiol., 95*, 431–441.

Oxley, D., Barrera, M., & Sadalla, E. (1981). Relationships among community size, mediators, and social support variables: A path analytic approach. *Am. J. Community Psychol., 9*, 637–651.

Parry, G., & Shapiro, D. (1986). Social support and life-events in working class women: Stress buffering or independent effects? *J. Arch. Gen. Psychiat., 43*, 315–323.

Pearlin, L. (1989). The sociological study of stress. *J. Health & Social Behav., 30*, 241–256.

Quittner, A., Glueckauf, R., & Jackson, D. (1990). Chronic parenting stress: Moderating versus mediating effect. *J. Personality and Soc. Psychol., 59*, 1266–1278.

Robles, T., & Klecolt-Glaser, J. (2003). The physiology of marriage: Pathways to health. *Physiology and Behavior, 79*, 409–416.

Rosen, L., & Moghadam, L. (1988). Social support, family separation, and well-being among military wives. *J. Behavioral Med., 14*, 64–70.

Ross, R., Altmaier, E., & Russell, D. (1989). Job stress, social support, and burn-out among counseling center staff. *J. Counseling Psychol., 36*, 464–470.

Roy, R. (2006). *Chronic Pain and Family: A Clinical Perspective.* New York. Springer.

Roy, R. (2007). Social dislocation and the chronic pain patient. In M. Bond (Ed.), *Encyclopedia of Pain.* Berlin, Heidelberg: Springer Verlag.

Tetzloff, C., & Barrera, M. (1987). Divorcing mothers and social support: Testing the specificity of buffering effects. *Am. J. Community Psychol., 15*, 419–434.

Thoits, P. (1982). Conceptual, methodological, and theoretical problems in studying social support as a buffer against life-stress. *J. Health and Social Behav., 23*, 145–159.

Uchino, B. (2006). Social support and health: A review of physiological proc-esses potentially underlying links to disease outcomes. *J. Behavioral Med., 29,* 377–387.

Wallston, B., Alagna, S., DeVellis, B., & DeVellis, R. (1983). Social support and physical health. *Health Psychology, 2*, 367–391.

Westman, M., Eden, D., & Shirom, A. (1985). Job, stress, cigarette smoking and cessation: The conditioning effects of peer support. *J. Soc. Sc. Med., 20*, 637–644.

Wilcox, B. (1981). Social support, life stress, and psychological adjustment: A test of buffering hypothesis. *Am. J. Community Psychol., 9*, 371–386.

Young, M., & Willmott, P. (1957). *Family and kinship and East London.* London: Routledge and Kegan Paul.

2 Chronic Childhood Physical Illnesses: Special Challenges

This chapter explores the impact of social support or lack thereof on children with physical illnesses. We recognize that the term physical illness covers an extraordinary array of conditions. However, our objective is to try and discern problems that may be common across the board. Factors such as the level of disability and parental health, and a multitude of others, influence the availability and effectiveness of social support. As will become evident as we progress through this chapter, parental – especially maternal – support is recognized as a key element in the support structure of the sick child. It is also widely acknowledged in the literature that the presence of a chronically ill child often exacts a heavy price on parental health and the healthy functioning of the family. Non-availability of resources has the potential to undermine the health of parents (Cohen, 1999). For a chronically sick child, parents often are the main source of support. Parents, however, experience strain and stress directly attributable to their parenting role, which creates a vicious cycle, thus making them vulnerable to morbidity.

Hence, the two interrelated issues are the extent to which parents maintain their health in the face of a potentially challenging situation (rearing a child with chronic physical illness) and their capacity to provide support for the affected child. To achieve our objectives we examine the research literature on the impact on parents' health and well-being, family function, and also the factors that protect them from negative consequences, in other words, their resiliency. Finally, we turn our attention to the central question of the buffering hypothesis of social support in relation to physically ill children.

Overview of the Problem

Childhood physical illnesses are widely prevalent. Juvenile Chronic Arthritis (JCA) alone, one of the most common childhood illnesses, has an estimated prevalence ranging from 0.16 to 1.13 cases per 1000 children (Benjamin, 1990). Between 30,000 and 50,000 children are diagnosed with Juvenile Rheumatoid Arthritis (JRA), the most common of JCA disorders, each year in the United States (Lawrence et al., 1998). When all the other relatively common childhood diseases such as asthma and diabetes are added together, the depth and breadth of the problem begin to loom large. About 5% of children in the Western world report persistent handicapping physical illness (Garralda, 1994). The most common illnesses are asthma, eczema, and epilepsy. Powerful evidence exists to show a link between severity of illness and psychiatric morbidity in children with chronic physical illnesses (ibid.). The diagnosis of a child with a chronic physical disease has the capacity to create considerable parental conflict and family dysfunction (Kazak, 1989). Mothers especially appear to be at risk, mainly due to the added responsibilities associated with raising a sick child (Noll et al., 1995; Silver et al., 1995). However, as Lazarus and Folkman (1984) observed, that stress is neither inherent in a situation nor solely attributable to an event such as chronic childhood illness. Rather, it is a product of person–environment interaction.

Parental Stress and Strain

Attachment is a key concept in our understanding of the mother/father–child relationship. Nedelisky (2004) conducted a comprehensive review of the literature on the impact of pediatric illness and disability on the attachment between child and parent (caregiver). She concluded that there was not much evidence to support a unidirectional causal relationship between chronic pediatric conditions and the quality of the child–caregiver attachment relationship. However, it was beyond question that the presence of such a child in a family may indeed constitute a risk factor for the child–caregiver attachment relationship. The point is that the cumulative influence of factors such as parental stress, depression, social isolation, and psychological maladjustment may very well have adverse impact on the child–parent attachment. It is a matter of common sense that the presence of a physically ill child in a family is likely to have an impact on parents' health and compromise their role as caregivers.

Manuel (2001) observed that the long-term effects could be as wide ranging as changes in family roles and patterns of intimacy, marital stress, and dysfunction. In short, parents' effectiveness as the main provider of support may be put in jeopardy. Mothers, in particular, tend to shoulder much of the responsibility for the sick child. The father's role is uncertain.

Sallfors and Hollberg (2003) found in their investigation of parental stress associated with raising a sick child that parents fulfilled differential roles in caring for the ill child. Mothers were more involved in every aspect of childcare and experienced 'intensive stress.' Several studies have reported on the psychological vulnerability of the mothers of chronic sick children (Eiser, 1990; Thompson and Gustafson, 1996; Timko, Stovel, and Moos, 1992). Fathers, by contrast, were found to be passive and waiting. An interesting finding was that the father's somewhat withdrawn and supportive role was for the 'well-being of the siblings and the whole family' (Sallfors & Hallberg, 2003).

An earlier study established a critical fact that the perceived well-being of the parents was directly associated with poorer adjustment of the children (Eiser, Haverman, Pancer, & Eiser, 1991). The subjects consisted of 287 mothers and 224 fathers. The children suffered from one of six conditions, namely, diabetes, asthma, epilepsy, leukemia, spina bifida, or cardiac disease. The goal of the study was to investigate age and gender differences in adjustment to chronic disease. The authors noted that mothers rated their children with leukemia and epilepsy as having greater difficulties, perhaps potentially reflecting a greater impact on normal life. Mothers also perceived these two groups as experiencing significant restrictions as a consequence of the disease. Mothers and fathers generally did not differ significantly in their perceptions. The most critical finding in this study was the recognition that parents' perceptions of the difficulties and restrictions associated with chronic disease were critical indices of their perceptions of children's adjustment. Parental perception could be an outcome of the distress associated with living with a seriously ill child.

Mohammed (2006) investigated maternal stress in a consecutive group of 64 mothers of children with intractable epilepsy in Jeddah, Saudi Arabia. In addition to a demographic and health questionnaire, a standardized fatigue scale that measured physical and mental fatigue was used. Most children, aged between one and fifteen years, had epilepsy for two years or more. Factors that contributed to increased maternal fatigue were the children's age (two years and under) and the physical status of the sick child, such as the type of epilepsy (cryptogenic) and severe motor deficits. Factors contributing to lower fatigue in the mothers were regular exercise, the absence of mental retardation in the children, and the lack of recent hospitalization. Mohammed noted that maternal fatigue may indeed affect the medical management of children, as it may compromise compliance with medication and confidence in the overall treatment. Furthermore, regular exercise and social support were recognized as key ingredients to maintains mothers' health and well-being.

The cost of family caregiving resulting in morbidity has the proportions of a major public health problem (McDaniel & Campbell, 1998). Parental coping is determined by a host of factors. Mothers with lower levels of social support and family cohesion demonstrate poorer levels of adjustment. Fathers with poor adjustment cope by trying to understand the child's medical situation, more family life-events and lower family cohesion (Dewey & Crawford, 2007). The presence of a sick child is likely to impact negatively on the health of the caregivers (parents) (Perez, 2007). In a controlled study of parents with and without asthmatic children, Perez concluded that caregivers without such children enjoyed better physical and mental health than caregivers with children who suffered from asthma.

The Perez paper illustrates in the most obvious way the impact of parental distress on the well-being of their children with juvenile rheumatoid disease (JRD) (Wagner, Chaney, Hommel, Page, et al. 2003). Subjects consisted of 45 children with JRA and their parents. Increased parental distress was significantly associated with greater child depressive symptomatology, demonstrating the transactional nature of child adjustment in childhood chronic illness. Parent distress had a significant impact on child depressive symptoms when children reported their illness as interfering with many aspects of their lives. The significance of the interaction of the parent-child variables was confirmed.

Our two final papers report on two important aspects of the intricate nature of the relationship between childhood chronic illness and parental health (Frankel & Wamboldt, 1998: Lopez, Mullins, Wolfe-Christensen, & Bourdeau, 2008). The direct relationship between a child's health and well-being and caregiver mental health was demonstrated in a study of 70 children with asthma and their caregivers, mostly mothers

(Frankel & Walmboldt, 1998). A variety of measures were used to assess children's mental status and parental and family functioning measures. The most important predictors of the level of impact a child's asthma had on the family were the level of reported emotional distress and the amount of social support the authors reported. The Parent's Psychiatric Symptoms Scale emerged as a powerful predictor of impact. Parents who demonstrated elevated levels of total emotional distress and low levels of perceived social support also reported a child's illness as disruptive and having significant impact on family life. Single parenthood was also associated with higher levels of distress. The reciprocal nature of stress in parents causing elevated distress in the children and vice versa was powerfully illustrated by this well-executed study.

Our final study also investigated the relation of perceived child vulnerability (PCV) and parental psychological distress (PPD) to adolescent anxiety (AANX) in youths with chronic illness (Lopez, Mullins, Wolfe-Christensen, & Bourdeau, 2008). Subjects consisted of 70 adolescents with either asthma or type 1 diabetes mellitus. Perceived PPD and PCV were major predictors of AANX. Although PPD was related to AANX, PCV accounted for a significant amount of variance in this relation. Parents who reported higher levels of psychological distress were more likely to perceive their child as vulnerable, which in turn could only add to the child's sense of vulnerability. Again the interrelatedness of parent-child distress and the reciprocal nature of this relationship received further confirmation.

Summary

The idea that, in the first place, a caregiver's health may be compromised by the stress of raising a chronically sick child and that, secondly, parental health, especially of mothers, may in turn have negative consequences for the child both lends itself to common sense and is supported by empirical evidence. Because of the intricate nature of this relationship, the preservation of parental health and morale must come under close scrutiny. However, Thompson and Gustafson (1996), following their most comprehensive review of this topic, concluded that studies that used structured diagnosis to assess parental distress were few and far between. Such information was usually based on self-reports generated by questionnaires. Nevertheless, they agreed that evidence suggested that parents and children with chronic illness themselves were at elevated risks for adjustment problems. The fact that many children and parents adapted successfully to a child's chronic illness was also undeniable.

The Chronically Sick Child and the Family

In this section we have included only studies with a control group and that used at least one measure to assess family functioning. In 2003 the Pediatric Task Force in the United States issued a report entitled 'Converging trends in family research and pediatrics: Recent findings for the American Academy of Pediatrics Task Force on the Family' (Wertlieb, 2003). In this sweeping report the task force covered almost every aspect of family issues as they impacted on pediatric research. The topics ranged from the relationship between marriage and the health of children to family religiosity and children's health. One observation directly relevant to this chapter was that children with married parents had an advantage in shaping their behaviour based on parental models that included behaviours such as compliance with a medical regimen, avoiding risk-taking behaviour, and leading a secure and scheduled lifestyle.

A major epidemiological investigation of the psychological adjustment of the parents of children with chronic illness provided a more comprehensive and complex view of this problem (Cadman, Rosenbaum, Boyle, and Offord, 1991). Mental health problems were two to three times higher in parents with chronically sick children compared to parents with healthy children. Some 29% of the mothers and 8% of the fathers with sick children reported mental health problems. Significantly, no differences emerged between groups in increases in single-parent families, social isolation, or alcohol problems. The authors concluded that there was no evidence to support the notion that families with chronically ill children functioned any differently than families without such children. Kazak (1992) compared families without children with physical disabilities with families with children with spina bifida, phenylketonuria, and mental retardation. A key finding was that parental stress was largely associated with the demands on parents related to the care of their children. Marital satisfaction remained unaffected. However, the level of parental stress could be significantly reduced by the presence of a social network that could provide emotional and material support, offer advocacy on behalf of parents, and help them with proper strategies for child-rearing (Cochran & Brassard, 1979)

Below we present a brief, wide-ranging review of the research literature on the relationship between psychological stress factors and asthma (Bloomberg and Chen, 2005). Bloomberg and Chen noted that non-compliance with the prescribed medication for children with asthma was often an indication of family conflict with biological consequences. Another factor that has a biological consequence may be related to family conflict, which has been demonstrated to affect the immune functioning of children. They further observed that families with limited psychological resources would have greater difficulty in effectively managing the child's illness well enough to avoid hospitalization or in predicting wheezing illness in infants. These findings show the potential harm that family dysfunction may have, not only for the psychological well-being, but also for the physical well-being, of a chronically sick child.

Complexities that surround the concept of the adjustment of sick children were addressed by Perrin and colleagues (1993) in an investigation of family and maternal influence on perceptions of adjustment. They investigated 187 children, including a control group and three groups of children with grand mal seizures, petit mal seizures, and visible conditions such as spina bifida and rheumatoid arthritis. Each child was assessed for psychosocial adjustment using standardized instruments. Parents' perspective and family functioning were captured by a number of valid instruments.

The results were complex. The authors noted that the relationship between a child's adjustment and health status was less than simple. Children's adjustment depended not only on their health status, but on their gender (girls were better adjusted), family environment, and, quite specifically, the mother's health locus of control, which meant that mothers who thought that they had greater control over their own health were likely to have similar feelings about their children's health. The quality of family life was found to have considerable impact on the children's psychosocial adjustment. This confirmed earlier studies that had shown that children who were better adjusted were likely to have families with high level of cohesion, well organized in their functioning, participating in outside social activities, and having the flexibility to modify family rules to accommodate the child. This was an important study, not only for its scope, but for the fact that it combined the child's environment (external factors) with the mother's health locus of control (an internal characteristic). The fact is that effective family functioning in the presence of a chronically sick child may present quite a challenge. And yet, we do find that many families show extraordinary resilience and continue to function at a high level. The following study attests to that.

Gerhardt and colleagues (2003) also concluded in their investigation of family functioning, among other factors, that families of children with Juvenile Rheumatoid Arthritis functioned at the same level as the matched control group of normal families. This study is carefully designed and well executed, and for that reason we will discuss it at some length. Subjects consisted of 64 children with JRA, 64 mothers and 46 fathers, along with 64 matched comparison families. The average duration of the JRA was 70 months. The goals of this study were to evaluate parental distress, family functioning, and social support among children with a lifetime diagnosis of rheumatoid arthritis. A number of standardized instruments were used to measure parental distress, family functioning, and social support.

The results showed that the JRA families and comparison families did not differ significantly on demographic factors. As for parental distress, no significant differences emerged between either group of mothers and fathers. Mothers were found to be similar in their level of distress, as were the fathers. However, further analysis of mothers who scored in the clinical range revealed that more mothers with JRA were in the clinical range (46%) than comparison mothers (28%). For fathers of children with JRA, 48% were in the clinical range, compared with 33% for the comparison fathers.

It was revealing that the clinical status of the mother of children with JRA was directly related to a number of factors associated with family functioning. Lower Supportive and higher Conflicted scores on the Family Environment Scale emerged as significant for the mother with JRA children. The family factors were not associated with the clinical status of the comparison group. Interestingly, on overall family functioning no significant differences emerged between the two groups.

On the critical issue of social support, the size of social support networks, and perceived functional support no significant differences were found between the JRA and the comparison groups. As for the impact on children, no significant associations emerged between parental distress, family functioning, or social support and the disease status of the children with JRA. The most telling conclusion of this study was that the families with JRA children demonstrated the same level of adjustment as those in the control group. Social support was not dissimilar for the two groups. Quite remarkably, disease factors such as severity, activity, and time since diagnosis did not show any association with the psychosocial variables. The authors offered two plausible explanations for these findings: (1) that these families were remarkably resilient in adapting to the demands of raising a chronically sick child or (2) that the parents did not find having such a child particularly challenging.

Our final paper in this section also investigated family and parental adjustment to chronic childhood disease. Subjects consisted of 20 mothers and 15 fathers of children with cystic fibrosis, 11 mothers and 9 fathers of children with muscular dystrophy, 18 mothers and 9 fathers of children with asthma, 13 mothers and 8 fathers of children with Type 1 diabetes, and 19 mothers and 11 fathers of healthy children (Dewey & Crawford, 2007). The major objective of this study was to determine the correlates of psychosocial adjustment to life-limiting and non-life-limiting chronic disease to assess if different factors were associated with maternal and paternal adjustment. Appropriate instruments were used to measure parental adjustment, family function, social support and coping strategies.

The findings revealed an interesting difference in the gender adjustment, as mothers reported significantly more difficulties than fathers. Family factors emerged as a major predictor for parental adjustment. Family cohesion was the most critical predictor for maternal adjustment. For fathers, family cohesion and total family life stress emerged as equally important predictors of adjustment. The most telling finding was the failure of the study to find any significant differences in the overall psychological functioning between parents of children with chronic disease and parents of healthy children. Another point of note was that being a stay-at-home parent seemed independent of whether the child had a disease or was healthy. It was not possible to compare two-parent families with single-parent ones due to their small numbers, but there was a suggestion that single-parent homes experienced a higher level of psychological distress than two-parent homes. It should be noted that this study did not provide any information on the impact of parental functioning on the health of the children. However, it would appear that given that parents with children with a disease functioned at the same level as parents with healthy children, it could be assumed that the children remained unaffected.

Summary

Many and varied factors influence a sick child's adjustment or non-adjustment. Perrin and colleagues (1993) found that family environment, the sick's child gender, and the mother's locus of control were all predictors of the child's adjustment, whereas Gerhardt and colleagues (2003), in their investigation of children with JRA, reached very different conclusions. No significant associations were found between parental distress, family environment, or social support and the disease status of the children. Dewey and Crawford (2007) failed to find any significant differences in the overall psychological functioning between parents of healthy and sick children. However, some family factors such as family cohesion were predictive of parental adjustment to having a chronically sick child. Different outcomes of these studies, in part, can be explained by the different children's populations, their health status, and the central goals of these studies. The impact of family and other factors on the children's adjustment was the objective of two of these studies (Gerhardt et al., 2003; Perrin et al., 1993). Dewey and Crawford (2007), by contrast, investigated parental adjustment. However, from a clinical point of view the healthy functioning of families with chronically sick children cannot be overemphasized. Parents in particular are the principal providers of support for children. Despite contradictory findings, it is reasonable to assume that compromised family functioning can have significant deleterious consequences for the sick children.

Social Support for Caregivers

The report of the American Academy of Pediatric Task Force on Project Resilience involved 124 families with a pre-adolescent child with a chronic illness or disability (Garwick, Patterson, Bennett, and Blum, 1998). One hundred and twenty-four parents were interviewed on their perception of social support in caring for their chronically sick children. Both fathers and mothers reported the importance of support from other family members. Support was both emotional and tangible. The parents appreciated the informational support they received from healthcare professionals.

Parents also commented on unhelpful support, much of which was from extended family members and sometimes healthcare professionals, which included rude or insensitive remarks. A one-year follow-up revealed a stable pattern of support. Authors concluded that the findings from this study suggested the significance of social support from wide-ranging sources, from extended family to healthcare professionals to schools. It was noteworthy that parents of these children received different types of support from various systems. Most critically, there was little overlap between the different kinds of support they received from differing sources. One noteworthy omission in this study was the impact of support or lack thereof on the children themselves.

The conclusion was that the 'social support system identified as emblematic of successful families to chronic illness can be measured and targeted for improving of care and quality of life.' The effectiveness of parenting a chronically sick child may be associated with a great many factors. It is noteworthy that chronic illness in the child enhances support in a number of social areas and promotes parent-child attachments in the absence of repeated potentially stressful separations. A child's illness has the potential of causing marital stress and even breakdown. However, there is also evidence to the contrary (Garralda, 1994). Garralda noted that many parents reported that a child's illness resulted in greater support. Many also reported that stress on their marriage and marital breakdown was, overall, not increased. Furthermore, she noted that chronic illness in a child may lead to heightened maternal empathy and sympathy towards the child. We noted in the preceding section that mothers with low levels of social support adjusted poorly to coping with chronically sick children.

Florian and Krulik (1991), in an early study of loneliness among mothers confronted with children with chronic life-threatening and non-threatening illness, investigated the value of social support. Subjects included 90 mothers, 33 of whom had a child with a life-threatening disease, and 57 had a child with a non-life-threatening chronic disease. The control group comprised 92 mothers with healthy children. Standardized loneliness and social support scales were used.

Apart from finding that mothers as the principal caregivers of children with a life-threatening disease experienced higher levels of loneliness than mothers of healthy children, results were complex in the sense that while greater social support was reported by the mothers of children with a life-threatening disease, no significant relationship emerged between the extent of social support and loneliness. An inverse relationship was found between social support and loneliness in both mothers with chronically sick children and the control group. Evidence was clear that while social support mitigated loneliness for mothers with chronically sick children, this was not true for mothers with children with a life-threatening disease. The authors offered a number of explanations for their findings. Among them, one that resonates is their observation that while mothers with chronic sick children may experience an overlap between social support and loneliness, for mothers of children with a life-threatening disease the two situations may not be interlinked. Furthermore, mothers of children with a life-threatening disease may be in a state of grief, which the authors describe as existential loneliness, and external social support plays little or no part in the mitigation of those feelings.

Summary

We are left with a complex picture. While social support was generally found to be useful in coping with a sick child, the type and quality of support also played a role. Marital stress was not a predictable feature, and the presence of a sick child also had the potential of strengthening the marital bond. Nevertheless, given the extent of parental, especially marital, distress associated with the presence of a sick child, social support may play a key role in maintaining parental health and well-being.

Social Support for Chronically Sick Children and the Buffering Hypothesis

In this final section we present a brief review of the literature directly addressing the beneficial effects of social support for children with chronic physical illness. We discuss two review articles addressing very different aspects of social support. We begin with a study that directly tested the hypothesis that social support moderated the effects of the micro-stressors (the buffering hypothesis) on the psychosocial adjustment of children with pediatric rheumatic disease (PRD) (von Weiss, Rapoff, Varni, Lindsay, et al., 2002).

Subjects in this study consisted of 160 children aged between 8 and 17. They were recruited from three pediatric rheumatology centres. In addition to demographic data, information related to disease severity, daily hassles, and social support was obtained using standardized measures. Additional data was collected on depression and anxiety in the children. One important finding was the affirmation of the main-effect model of social support. Data failed to support the buffering relationship between daily hassles, adjustment, and social support. However, certain kinds of social support, such as from classmates and parents, proved to be the best predictors of adjustment relative to friend or teacher support. This study had many strengths, such as the number of sites from which the subjects were chosen, multiple measures of adjustment for parents and children, and a larger sample size compared to previous studies. Targeting classmate and parental support to improve the functioning of children with PRD was recommended. The buffering hypothesis received , if at all, only nominal validation.

In a major review of the social support and adolescent cancer-survivor literature, Decker (2007) noted many shortcomings in the research methodologies employed by many investigations. The sample size in many of these studies was small, which made it difficult to gauge the true effect size due to low power. Decker expressed particular concern with a lack of consistency in the conceptualization and measurement of social support. While childhood cancer is outside the scope of this chapter, we chose to include this particular review because the focus was on survivors and because of the similarity of findings with other chronic childhood disorders.

Altogether seventeen studies included in Decker's review were basically descriptive and exploratory in nature. Only eight studies examined social support in relation to a number of outcome variables. One finding supported the observation that support from friends was not necessarily effective and was less so than parental, especially maternal, support. This is despite the fact that friends were considered to be 'extremely' important. Support from parents, while critical, was not without its problems. Many adolescents found it difficult to spend a lot of time with the family, and they often felt that their privacy was being compromised. Support from healthcare professionals was not systematically investigated. However, Decker concluded that social support from friends and classmates facilitated the adolescents' disease adaptation and could help with the lifestyle aspects of treatment regimen. This review is of particular importance because it identified major methodological issues that continue to beset social-support outcome research.

Our final review of reviews reported on the role of peers and close friend in reducing health risks in children and adolescents with chronic physical illness (LaGreca, Bearman, & Moore, 2002). The purpose of this review was to answer three questions: (1) the role of peers and close friends as a source of support for youth with pediatric conditions; (2) friends' influence in treatment adherence; and (3) peers' and friends' impact on health-promoting and health-risk behaviours. Findings were varied and complex. Types of disease influenced outcome in relation to all three areas of influence. In relation to the first, there was evidence that support from close friends and family members lowered levels of behavioural problems compared to children with support from only one source. In certain conditions, however, such as Type 1 diabetes, research showed that friends were a more powerful source of support than parents. Self-disclosure to a close friend could be a source of support. However, with more visible conditions, medical explanation to classmates may negatively influence their response.

As for treatment adherence, friends could be a source of support with conditions such as diabetes. One problem identified was non-compliance on the part of the children and adolescents to avoid calling attention to themselves. The role of peers and friends in promoting health and avoiding risky behaviours could be very complex. With behaviours such as smoking, drug and alcohol use, and risky social behaviour, research findings were inconclusive. The reviewers noted that how peers affected the health-risk behaviours of children with chronic illness, while very important, was under-researched.

The conclusion of this review was that children with chronic illness demonstrated a high level of resiliency and that these children have comparable peer relationships to their healthy counterparts. Children with visible health problems were likely to encounter problems in their peer relationships. Friends did serve as a major source of emotional support.

Summary

The buffering role of social support for chronically sick children is an inconclusive matter, and results are mixed. There is some consensus that social support, on the whole, is beneficial from many different perspectives. Yet, Decker's (2007) paper raises very important questions about the buffering effect, which she found to be elusive due to a host of methodological problems. Even with that limitation, social support proved beneficial in diverse situations. LaGreca and her associates (2002) were less concerned about the methodological issues. Nor did they describe their criteria for the inclusion of articles in their review, which lacked the rigour of the review paper by Decker. Nevertheless, the buffering hypothesis did receive support in their review. The visibility of a child's condition was a determining factor so far as peer support was concerned. Von Weiss and colleagues (2002) reported an unambiguous benefit of classmate support in mitigating depression in children with rheumatic disease. The buffering hypothesis was not supported by this particular study. The most general conclusion that can be drawn is that the presence of social support for children with chronic illness is, on the whole, beneficial. Its actual power seems dependent on a host of factors. The buffering hypothesis remains somewhat elusive.

Conclusion

In this chapter we have tried to present a synopsis of a vast and complicated topic, and in that process we might have excluded issues that may be seen as critical. We acknowledge the possibility of such omission. Our overarching conclusion, setting aside the debate between the main effects of social support vis-à-vis the buffering hypothesis, is that social support of many kinds serves crucial functions in promoting more effective coping in diverse areas of functioning. Parents, especially mothers, play a crucial role as a central source of support for a chronically sick child. However, the stress and strain associated with child-care also makes them vulnerable to morbidity. Equally, such variables as the severity and visibility of the disease influence the benefits that may accrue for effective social support. Parents, close friends, classmates, and peers all play a role in helping the children manage their disease with greater resiliency.

REFERENCES

Benjamin, C. (1990). Review of UK data on the rheumatic diseases – 1. Juvenile chronic arthritis. *Br. J. Rheumatology, 29*, 231–233.
Bloomberg, G., & Chen, E. (2005). The relationship of psychologic stress with childhood asthma. *Immunol. Allergy Clin. North Am., 25*, 83–105.
Cadman, D., Rosenbaum, P., Boyle, M., & Offord, D. (1991). Children with chronic illness: Family and parent demographic characteristics and psychosocial adjustment. *Pediatrics, 87*, 884–889.
Cochran, M., & Brassard, J. (1979). Child development and personal social network. *Child Development, 50*, 601–616.
Cohen, M. (1999). Families coping with chronic childhood illnesses: A research review. *Families, Systems, and Health, 17*, 149–164.
Decker, C. (2007). Social support and adolescent cancer survivors: A review of the literature. *Psycho-Oncology, 16*, 1–11.
Dewey, D., & Crawford, S. (2007). Correlates of maternal and paternal adjustment to chronic childhood disease. *J. Clin. Psychol. Medical Settings, 14*, 219–226.

Eiser, C. (1990). *Chronic childhood disease: An introduction to psychological theory and research*. Cambridge: Cambridge University Press.

Eiser, C., Havermans, T., Pancer, M., & Eiser, R. (1991). Adjustment to chronic disease in relation to age and gender: Mothers' and fathers' reports of their children's behavior. *J. Pediat. Psychol., 17*, 261–275.

Florian, V., & Krulik, T. (1991). Loneliness and social support of mothers of chronically ill children. *Soc. Sc. Med., 32*, 1291–1296.

Frankel, K., & Wamboldt, M. (1998). Chronic childhood illness and maternal mental health: Why should we care? *J. Asthma, 35*, 621–630.

Garralda, M. (1994). Chronic physical illness and emotional disorder in childhood: Where the brain is not involved, there may still be problems. *Br. J. Psychiatry, 164*, 8–10.

Garwick, A., Patterson, J., Bennett, F., & Blum, R. (1998). Parents' perception of helpful vs unhelpful types of support in managing the care of preadolescents with chronic conditions. *Arch. Pediat. & Adolescent Med., 152*, 1–13.

Gerhardt, C., Vannatta, K., McKellop, J., Zeller, M., et al. (2003). Comparing parental distress, family functioning, and the role of social support for caregivers with and without a child with juvenile rheumatoid arthritis. *J. Pediat. Psychol., 28*, 5–15.

Kazak, A. (1989). Families of chronically ill children: A systems and social-ecological model of adaptation and challenge. *J. Consul. Clin. Psychol., 57*, 25–30.

Kazak, A. (1992). The social context of coping with childhood chronic illness: Family systems and social support. In A. LaGreca, L. Siegel, J. Wallander, & C. Walker (Eds.), *Advances in pediatric psychology: Stress and coping with pediatric conditions* (pp. 262–278). New York: Guilford.

LaGreca, A., Bearman, K., & Moore, H. (2002). Peer relations of youth with pediatric conditions and health risks: Promoting social support and healthy lifestyles. *J. Developmental Behavioral Pediatrics, 23*, 271–280.

Lawrence, R., Helmick, C., Arnett, F., Deyo, R., et al. (1998). Estimates of the prevalence of arthritis and selected musculoskeletal disorders in the United States. *Arthritis & Rheumatism, 41*, 778–799.

Lazarus, R., & Folkman, S. (1984). *Stress, appraisal and coping*. New York: Springer.

Lopez, W., Mullins, L., Wolfe-Christensen, C., & Bourdeau, T. (2008). The relation between parental psychological distress and adolescent anxiety in youths with chronic illness: The mediating effect of perceived child vulnerability. *Children's Health Care, 37*, 171–182.

Manuel, J. (2001). Risk and resistance factors in the adaptation in mothers of children with juvenile chronic arthritis. *J. Pediat. Psychol., 22*, 237–246.

McDaniel, S., & Campbell, T. (1998). Family caregiving and coping with chronic illness (editorial). *Family, Systems, and Health, 16*, 195–196.

Mohammed, J. (2006). Intractable childhood epilepsy and maternal fatigue. *Can. J. Neurological Sciences, 33*, 306–310.

Nedelisky, A. (2004). Attachment relationships between children with physical disabilities and their caregivers. *Graduate Students J. Psychology, 6*, 5–12.

Noll, R., Garstein, M., Hawkins, A., Vannatta, K , et al. (1995). Comparing parental distress for families with children who have cancer and matched comparison families without children. *Fam. Sys. Med., 13*, 11–28

Perez, P. (2007). The relationship between childhood asthma status and caregiver health outcome. *Dissertation Abstracts International*, section B: The Sciences and Engineering, *68* (4-B).

Perrin, E., Ayoub, C., & Willett, J. (1993). In the eye of the beholder: Family and maternal influence on perceptions of adjustment of children with a chronic illness. *Developmental and Behavioral Pediatrics, 14*, 94–105.

Sallfors, C., & Hallberg, L. (2003). A parental perspective on living with a chronically ill child: A qualitative study. *Families, Systems, and Health, 21*, 193–204.

Silver, E., Bauman, L., & Ireys, H. (1995). Relationships of self-esteem and efficacy to psychological distress in mothers of children with chronic physical illness. *Health Psychology, 6*, 333–340.

Thompson, R., & Gustafson, K. (1996). *Adaptation to chronic childhood illness*. Washington, DC: American Psychological Association.

Timko, C , Stovel, K., & Moos, R. (1992). Functioning among mothers and fathers of children with juvenile rheumatic disease. *J. Pediat. Psychol., 6*, 705–724.

Von Weiss, R., Rapoff, M., Varni, J., Lindsley, C., Olson, N., et al. (2002). Daily hassles and social support as predictors of adjustment in children with pediatric rheumatic disease. *J. Pediatric Psychol., 27*, 155–165.

Wagner, J., Chaney, J., Hommel, K., Page, M., et al. (2003). The influence of parental distress on child depressive symptoms in juvenile rheumatic disease: The moderating effect of illness intrusiveness. *J. Pediat. Psychol., 28*, 453–462.

Wertlieb, D. (2003). Converging trends in family research and pediatrics: Recent findings for the American Academy of Pediatrics on the family. *Pediatrics, 111*, 1572–1582.

3 Spousal and Long-Term Partnership Support: How Critical Is It?

In the preceding chapter, the key role of the mother as the main caregiver and source of support for a chronic sick child was established beyond doubt. This chapter begins with a brief exploration of the value of spousal support in the care of a chronically sick partner, which is empirically demonstrated to produce many positive outcomes. The rest of the chapter is devoted to an analysis of the current state of marriage and the family at the onset of a new century, and its implications for family and spouse as sources of social support.

Spouse/Partner and Social Support

It must be acknowledged at the outset that the research literature on marriage and social support is huge, and our limited purpose in this section is to provide a brief overview of this topic. Brown and Harris, in their seminal work (1978) on depression in community-living women, were able to confirm a common-sense observation that the availability of an intimate or confidante reduced risk factors for depression after the experience of negative life-events or even persistent difficulties. Availability of a partner was considered the highest category of support. McFarlane and colleagues (1983) reported on the nature of social support based on a longitudinal study to investigate the relationship between stress and morbidity and two factors, namely, social support and locus of control that mediated the relationship. The findings were complicated, but one particular outcome confirmed a long-standing view that intimate relations played a powerful role in maintaining health or mitigating stress. The researchers found that 'helpfulness of social supports was causally related to the occurrence of stressful evens, so that an individual with helpful social support was less likely to experience stressful events' and 'individuals who report smaller but overall more effective networks also report that their inner core of intimates are considerably more helpful' (p. 171). The intimates, generally speaking, are usually spouses or partners.

Spousal role in the mitigation of disease continues to be a major focus of research. Thoits (1995), in an exhaustive review of the role of social support and stress, concluded that intimate, confiding relationships are those that best confer the beneficial effects of social support. Intimate and confiding relationships, while not confined to marriage or a partnership, are more likely to be found in a long-term partner/marriage relationship.

While there is wide acceptance of the value of spousal support, the following study expanded on the theme by examining the effectiveness of a past peer mentoring experience (PME) as well as a current live-in partner (LIP) with 62 individuals with spinal cord injury (SCI) (Sherman and DeVinney, 2004). On average, SCI subjects had lived with their injury for 11.7 years. Different types of support yielded different benefits. A PME that had terminated over 10 years ago was associated with higher occupational activity and life-satisfaction. LIP, by contrast, promoted greater mobility and economic independence.

The authors provided several possible explanations for the findings, ranging from the fact that those who benefited from PME were more competent and would have done well regardless or to the fact that they were fortunate to find an understanding and sympathetic peer. As for LIP, authors noted that greater life-satisfaction and financial security led to contact with peers, but not vice versa. This study provided somewhat indirect support for McFarlane et al's (1983) finding that those who had intimate relationships also enjoyed a larger social network. Sherman and DeVinney's (2004) study is instructive, as it demonstrates, and this is well documented in research, that spousal support alone was not sufficient, although it could be a prerequisite for effective coping.

The following study adopted a very different approach to the value of partner support by exploring the absence of such support for 219 women with early stage of breast cancer (Manne, Ostroff, Winkel, Grana, & Fox, 2005). A strong correlation was found between patient and partner ratings of unsupportive behaviour. Such behaviour, on the part of both, predicted more avoidant coping and distress. A patient's perception mediated the association between their partner's ratings of unsupportive behaviour and patient distress. The results were unambiguous in showing the negative consequences of unsupportive partner behaviour on the quality of life of women with early-stage breast cancer. This study provided negative evidence of the downside of unsupportive intimate relations.

The following points are noteworthy. First, the findings suggested that partner ratings of unsupportive behaviour and women's avoidant coping and distress were largely explained by women's perception of their partners' behaviour. This seemed to indicate that women's perception of their partners' behaviour had detrimental consequences. Furthermore, the results demonstrated a longitudinal association between unsupportive partner behaviours and avoidant coping and distress. It is equally noteworthy that unsupportive partner behaviour did not have any negative consequences unless the woman perceived the behaviours as unsupportive. The perception of unsupportive behaviour may have the same consequences as the absence of support, or perhaps could be worse. That remains an open question. This study highlighted the importance of the quality of communication and its consequences, which has broad clinical significance.

Our next report explored in a longitudinal study the effects of social support and personal coping resources on depressive symptoms in older patients with no chronic disease or with recently symptomatic diabetes mellitus, lung disease, cardiac disease, arthritis, or cancer. (Penninx, van Tilburg, Boeke, Deeg, et al., 1998). A sample of older persons between the ages of 55 and 85 was randomly drawn from population registers in the Netherlands. The final sample comprised 2810 persons. Information was gathered on disease status, social support, and personal coping resources.

The findings were complicated, but the buffering hypothesis received some degree of validation. Two buffer effects were found. For relationships that were considered 'diffused,' negative associations were found in relation to diabetes mellitus, lung disease, arthritis, and cancer. Emotional support and diffuse relationships interacted with specific diseases predicting depressive symptoms. Curiously, receiving instrumental support was predictive of depressive symptoms. Buffer effects were differential across diseases for emotional support (in cardiac disease and arthritis) and for diffuse relationships (in lung disease). It is also worthy of attention that the favourable effects of having a partner and many close relationships represented direct effects, as they seemed to occur regardless of the presence of chronic disease. Authors noted that this particular finding confirmed an observation made by Cohen and

Wills (1985) that direct health effects were generally found when structural support measures were used, whereas buffer effects were associated with the use of functional measures. This study revealed why it may be necessary to consider specific aspects of a patient's situation in order to have a better understanding about why some coping resources are more effective in one specific chronic disease than in another.

Our final two reports address two not too frequently discussed issues in the social support literature. Harrison and colleagues (1995) explored the gender issues as they pertain to confiding, and Coyne and DeLongis (1986) examined the positive and negative aspect of marriage as they pertain to social support.

Harrison and colleagues began by acknowledging the inherent value of social support in mitigating stress. They undertook a study to rectify an oversight that they claimed had been persistent in the social support literature, namely, gender bias. The majority of research had focused exclusively on women, despite evidence that major differences could be observed in the way men and women utilized social support. They interviewed a consecutive series of 520 subjects within a framework of eight weeks of a cancer diagnosis. The age range of the subjects was 17–75. There were 129 males and 391 females. Of these, 93 males and 255 females were either married or cohabiting. The diagnosis of cancer comprised breast, bowel, gynecological, lymphoma, and testicular.

Confiding behaviour was classified in two categories: no/little confiding and mainly fully confiding. Subjects were compared according to the degree of confiding their main concerns. 45% of men reported using only one confidante, compared to only 25% of women. Because three of the diseases were gender-specific, only two diseases, lymphoma and bowel cancer, were used for comparing the pattern of confiding between the genders. For lymphoma, more men (28%) than women (13%) confided in one person, and 27% men confided in their partners versus only 7% of women. For bowel cancer, more men (60%) used one confidante than did women (27%). Again, more men used partners than did women. Unfortunately, this study did not investigate the buffering effects of the supportive relationships. The authors noted the striking differences between men and women in the use of confidantes when faced with a potentially serious medical challenge. Contrary to general belief, men were able to use confiding relationships more than the female patients.

We end this section on a cautionary note. Coyne and DeLongis (1986) drew attention to the specifics of marriage as a source of social support.

Marriage may or may not be a happy state of affairs, and that would determine the presence or absence of support within the relationship. They also discussed the relevance of social support to clinical intervention, a subject we discuss in chapter 9. In this sweeping paper, the consequences of the lack of social support, marriage and social support, the negative side of social relationships, and the role of perceived support were examined.

The authors challenged the 'common' perception that married persons were generally healthier and happier. One key question they raised was whether, in the face of stress, support from other relationships might compensate for an unhappy marriage. The weight of research suggested that an alternative confiding relationship did not sufficiently offset the benefits of a confiding marital relationship. Besides, there was evidence to the effect that the group that was best off had a confiding marital relationship regardless of the presence or absence of a confiding relationship outside the marriage. A spouse/partner as a source of social support was not easily replaceable.

Summary

There is significant evidence that spousal/partner social support has a powerful buffering effect. Effective social support reducing the risk for morbidity from stressful events, a relationship between intimate relationship and a larger network of social support, the consequences of unsupportive partner behaviour, the differential buffering effects of a partner relationship in older adults with chronic disorders, the role of gender in seeking intimate partner support behaviour, and the complications associated with marriage, which in itself could be stressful, is but a short list of the scrutiny that marital/partner and social support research has come under. In broad terms, research has confirmed the main effects and/or buffering effect of a partner relationship that is stable, reciprocal, and intimate in the face of stressful events or situations. We noted the role of the mother in moderating the negative consequences of pediatric disease in their children. In the section above, the power of the significance of a partner relationship as a major factor in the mitigation of stress was discussed. In view of the value of family relationships, we now turn our attention to the state of the family in Canada in particular and the West in general. Two questions we try to answer are, What may be the risks associated with single parenthood, and Is marriage or a long-term relationship necessarily a predictor of good health?

What Is a Family?

An overview: In the preceding sections, the value of marriage and family as a central source of social support received a high level of validation. What is the current state of family at this point in history? The truth, however, is that in contemporary Western society there exist a plethora of family types, some of which were simply beyond our comprehension not so long ago. Divorce, which in the 1950s and 1960s was an aberration or exception to the general rule, is now considered a normally occurring event. Over the last thirty years or so the institution of the family has undergone a kind of transformation which is unparalleled in our history. Is the institution of the family under siege? Is the family as a source of social and emotional support in some peril? In the following pages we provide an overview of the current state of the family in the West. With a rising number of single-person households and single parents, is the availability of one of the key sources of social support, namely, intimate, supportive, and reciprocal partner relationships at risk, thus placing a significant proportion of the population in some jeopardy if and when they confront stressful situations.

In a recent television program on the Canadian Broadcasting Corporation (26 February 2009) entitled 'Bio-Dad,' the story of a gay man with a child was presented. This child and his gay father constituted a kind of family that might have been inconceivable a few short years ago. The child was conceived by artificial insemination. In fact, a single, gay man with a child is such a recent phenomenon that there is no recognition of it in the Canadian census of 2006. This program told the story of a man who was a product of artificial insemination, and his quest to find the identity of his biological father. In the process, he discovered several half-siblings. He eventually did learn the identity of his father. A time might come when it will be possible for two people of the same gender to have a biological child. We tell this story simply to illustrate that the common assumption behind the word 'family' is gone. The nuclear family is now a minority phenomenon in the scheme of family types.

The nuclear family, consisting of two biological parents and children, is now in a minority position in the Western world. In the United Kingdom, the nuclear family declined from 31% to 21% of family types between 1971 and 2000 (BBC Online Health, 2001). The 2006 Canadian census reported that the proportion of families with mother, father, and children was on the decline compared to couples with no children. However, parents with children continue to be the largest group. Between 1981 and 2001 the proportion of common-law families more than doubled from 6 to 14%. Another point of note was that a growing number of children were living in 'other' types of family structures. In 2001 a full 13% (732,900) of children 14 and under were living with parents in a common-law relationship. Another 12% lived with blended families (Statistics Canada, 2006b). According to the 2006 census, Canada had 45,350 same-sex couples. Of these 24,740 were male and 20,610 female. Marriage among the same-sex couples was less common (7460) versus common-law relationships (37,885). The number of children living with same-sex couples was not reported.

The most telling development that has significantly contributed to the decline of nuclear families is the rise of single-person households. According to the 2006 Canadian census, of 12,437,500 households, 26.8% were single-person households. In 1941, this figure was only 6%. In 2006, 27.1% of the households in United States were single-person, in Norway, 38.5%, in New Zealand, 22.6%, and Australia, 20.7%. In Great Britain one-person households increased from 23% in 1979 to 32% in 2000 (Walker et al., 2001–2). Households also have been steadily declining in size as people have fewer children or no children living at home (Statistics Canada, 2006a). Another clear trend is that fewer and fewer people are getting married. Only 20 years ago 61.4% of the population over the age of 15 were married. In 2006 that figure declined to 48.5% (Statistics Canada, 2006b). Advances in reproductive technology and genetics, combined with major changes in societal values over the last three decades, have produced these far-reaching changes in family structure.

The Perils of Single Parenthood

The single-parent family, on the rise for the last two decades, has many faces. An astonishing fact to come out of the 2006 census was the precipitous rise of unmarried single parents (Statistics Canada, 2006b). Nearly 30% of the single parents were never married, while 19% were widowed. At the middle of the last century, only 3.1% single parents were unmarried. Single parenthood does not constitute a single group. While this phenomenon seems to predominate in the poorer segment of society, other forms of single-parent families have emerged over the past few decades. Professional unmarried women are having children by choice. Yet, divorce is a major contributory factor. Nearly 30% of single parents were divorced (Statistics Canada, 2006b).

In this context an Irish study is worthy of our attention (McCashin, 1996). Ireland during the 1990s shed its image as a European economic and even social backwater and emerged as the Celtic Tiger. This miraculous economic ascendency also produced vast social changes. A prominent Irish social scientist, McCashin captured the nature of the changing society in his in-depth analysis of the emerging phenomenon of single parenthood by probing into the lives of some 53 single mothers in an area near Dublin. In 1981 only 5.7% (23,684) of the families with at least one child were lone mothers. By 1986, this had risen to 7.2% (30,568), an increase of 29.1%. Between 1986 and 1991, the proportion of single-mother households had risen to 9.9% (38,235), an increase of 25.1% from 1986.

McCashin identified an important element related to single parenthood, which was the degree to which women 'chose to be single mothers' (p. 186). Based on in-depth interviews, the author was impressed by the determination of these women to terminate a bad marriage and at the same time retain control of the children. The women enjoyed the experience of daily independence and their enhanced opportunities for personal growth and financial independence. However, this autonomy took place in the context of poverty. Many of these women lived in relative poverty in a country with ever-rising income and expectation. Social support was available to some of these young women (11/53) who lived with their parents. This support, however, was often negated by family conflicts and a desire for independence. Loneliness was expressed as a common experience by the single parents. McCashin's book is an exploration into the condition and social needs of single mothers. The focus is on social policy that would create social assets to enable these women to counteract some of the negative consequences of living in poverty.

At the outset of this section we gave an account of a single gay man with a child. Unfortunately, the 2006 census did not provide any information on the gender of the single parents. However, fathers also find themselves heading these families. What their proportion might be is not reported in the 2006 census. The problems associated with single parenthood are well understood. Yet, there is no cohesive social policy to adequately address their concerns.

Many of the problems we associate with single parenthood are rooted in poverty. There is also mounting evidence that children of divorced parents are also at higher risk for a variety of problems. Single parents in many Western countries are among the poorest. We focus on two aspects: first, the health risks associated with single parenthood, and second, depression in this population.

Health Risks

Single parents, especially mothers who also happen to be, more often than not, poor, are frequently at risk for multiple health and social prob-lems. There are, however, contradictory findings about the health risks associated with single parenthood. Harris and colleagues (1999), in a methodologically sound study, investigated family coping with type 1 diabetes mellitus (DM1) in intact, blended, and single-parent families. Data on wide-ranging medical, social, and psychological factors were collected from 119 adolescents (average age 14.3 years) and their pri-mary caregivers. Sixty-five adolescents came from intact families, 38 from single-parent families, and 16 from blended families.

These three types of families did not show any significant differences in the understanding of their children's functioning. Nevertheless, on some key issues the families functioned quite differently. One worri-some finding was that children from single-parent families, especially African American, had measurably poorer metabolic control. One plau-sible explanation for this finding was ineffectual parenting. The authors concluded that family composition, in itself, was not a reliable predic-tor of health outcome. Specific family factors had to be the focus of future research.

Large-scale population-based studies of single parents tend to pro-duce a rather gloomy picture. A Swedish study found that, compared with mothers in partnership, single mothers had a 70% increased risk of early death (Ringsback, Haglund, & Rosen, 2000). It was not just the single mothers who were at higher risk of early death; so were their offspring (Sauvola, Rasanen, Joukamaa, Jokelainen, et al., 2000). This Finnish population study was based on a prospectively collected birth cohort of 12,058 live births, which covered 96% of all children born in northern Finland in 1966. The cohort members' family background was assessed in 1980. At that time 19% lived in single-parent families.

Of the total cohort, 117 individuals died between the ages of 16 and 28. The overall mortality rate for the males was three times higher than for females. Further analysis showed that the mortality rates for males from single-parent families was significantly higher than for two-par-ent families. The highest risk increase was related to suicides. One plau-sible explanation for this finding was that there is increased risk for depression among people who experienced parental loss in childhood. Furthermore, affective disorders increased the risk of suicide.

One German study based on a review of the pertinent literature of the previous fourteen years, reported that 2.4 million lone parents with children were living in Germany in 2003 (Neises & Gruneberg, 2005). Over 80% of them were women. This study noted that the single parents were beset by low income, unemployment, and dependency on social welfare, which all produced a negative effect on the health outcomes of the parents as well as their children.

As for health outcomes, the reviewers arrived at a stark conclusion that mothers bringing up children alone tended to be more vulnerable to chronic disease than their married counterparts with children. This phenomenon seemed to be common across national boundaries. Similar findings were confirmed in England, Canada, the Netherlands, Australia, and Sweden. Sweden, which enjoys extensive state-based benefits, had the same problem with single mothers. A rather telling conclusion reached by this review was that unfavourable health outcomes were not necessarily a function of single parenthood. Rather, poverty, poor education, many offspring, and a dependency on state welfare, combined with poor utilization of healthcare services, accounted for poorer health outcomes than with their married counterparts. The children of single parents were also more vulnerable to poverty and illness. The authors recommended that in order to measure the impact of socio-economic factors on the health of single parents, future studies should focus on subgroups such as poor single parents, financially secure single parents, poor married parents and financially secure married parents.

In a survey of British and Swedish households, Whitehead and colleagues (2000) reviewed data spanning 1975 to 1995. Lone mothers in both countries had significantly worse health than their married counterparts, and the difference, surprisingly, was more or less of the same magnitude. This was an unexpected finding in view of the dramatically lower rates of poverty experienced by single mothers in Sweden, which was a direct consequence of progressive social policies. Further analysis showed that the health risks associated with poverty did not necessarily account for the different outcomes in the two countries.

The role of poverty was shown in a comparative study of Canada and Norway (Curtis and Phipps, 2004). Canadian single mothers had a significantly worse state of health than married mothers. This was not true in Norway, one explanation being that while both countries were similarly wealthy, single mothers in Canada faced greater threats of becoming poor and dependent on social welfare. The relationship between poverty and health was in the predictable direction.

The authors conducted a simulation to determine the estimated marginal effects associated with moving individuals from the lowest category into the second lowest category. This meant moving 97% of the mothers in the lowest category to the next highest income category, with the predicted result of a significant increase in health status. This did not prove to be the case. The pathways between income and health are complex, and simply raising the income alone could not accomplish that goal. The authors concluded that Norway had a social support system which was absent in Canada, including day care, days off for sick children, long and flexible maternity/parental leaves, and more. Here was some evidence that institutional social support, beyond partner support, had the potential of reducing health risks. It also confirmed our earlier observation that varying circumstances call for differing support systems.

Another Canadian population-based study found that single parenthood, maternal depression, and poverty were the major predictors for pediatric hospitalization (Guttmann, Dick, & To, 2004). Low-income adequacy or single parenthood increased the risk of hospitalization for a child one and a half times. Maternal depression emerged as the most powerful predictor of infant hospitalization. Curiously, the most powerful factor that protected a child from hospitalization was having either parent be a recent immigrant to Canada. Another curious finding was that the hospitalized group was significantly less likely to have a working mother. Did depression and poverty coexist in this population?

Nevertheless, while single parenthood emerged as a risk factor, maternal depression was the most powerful predictor of infant hospitalization. Maternal depression, at least in this study, superseded the buffering effect of being married. Data for this study was drawn from the Canadian National Longitudinal Survey of Children and Youth Cycle 1, collected in 1994–5. Only infants aged between 12 and 24 months were included. The final cohort consisted of 2184 infants. This study identified the vulnerability of single mothers in one specific domain of child-rearing.

Summary

The term 'family' has lost its singular meaning. In popular language family continues to be associated with the nuclear family. Yet the nuclear family has been on the decline for more than four decades. The single-person household is on the rise. The blended family is common. Add to that families with adopted children, common-law relations, single parents (ranging from teenagers to divorced adults, to individuals choosing to have a child in the absence of a partner, to a single gay parent), families with an artificially inseminated parent/child, gay couples with and without children, and we begin to appreciate the magnitude of this change. Societally and politically, these changes are far reaching and have serious policy implications. The latter, however, is beyond the scope of our current undertaking.

One point of note is that there does not seem to be any direct evidence to suggest that the absence of the buffering/main effect for single parents is directly attributable to their plight; only that divorce and separation often have an impact on the income of single mothers, not infrequently reducing them to poverty. Depression in the children of single parents was, however, attributed to the absence of a father, which the researchers claimed was rooted in the break-up of the marriage. Poverty is one factor for poorer health and even premature mortality, but that may provide only a partial explanation for the risk factors associated with single parenthood. As was noted, a general lack of social assets, such as day care, training programs, flexible working hours, and state income above the poverty line may all mitigate the ill effects of single parenthood.

Single Parenthood and Depression

We now examine in a very broad sense one of the more common conditions associated with single parenthood, depression. We present only a selected review of population-based studies, focusing on recent literature.

Poverty among single parents is highly predictable of depression. This is an important perspective, because social support in itself may not be the single most critical factor to mitigate depression in this population. Brown and Moran (1997) reported on 404 mothers with a child living at home. Single mother constituted 25% of the total sample. Their report is based on a two-year follow-up, during which period 117 women spent time as a single mother. Financial hardship was particularly common in single mothers. A third of the single mothers reported financial hardship during the initial interview. A point of note is that the risk of an onset of depression was high among single mothers irrespective of financial hardship. Negative experiences such as humiliation/entrapment events were much higher among them than for married mothers. The length of single parenthood was not a significant factor. Employment emerged as a significant factor for working single mothers (38%) compared to the rest (14%). Most reported enjoying their full-time jobs, but the cost was high. They were generally tired and concerned about possible neglect of their children. A most noteworthy factor was that very few mothers developed depression without psychological risk factors such as a negative environment (poor interpersonal relationships) and negative evaluation of self (poor self-esteem). This study contributed significantly to our understanding of the sources of depression in single mothers.

A Belgian study found an unequivocal relationship between 'ceasing to live with a partner' (relationship breakdown) and depression (Lorant, Croux, Weich, Deliege, et al., 2007). The sample consisted of 11,909 individuals, each of whom participated in an average 4.6 waves (times), providing 54,941 observations. A change in poverty and subjective financial strain had a greater effect on women than men. Women were more susceptible to developing depression than men. Ceasing to cohabit with a partner was a significant risk factor, particularly among women. On the other hand, embarking on a cohabiting relationship reduced depression more among women than in men. The value of an intimate relationship in mitigating depression was implied in this study. The authors cautioned that their results supported the notion that risk of depression was not a result of personal vulnerability or lack of resilience. This study did not provide any data on the family composition of the subjects.

A Canadian population-based study confirmed that mothers making a transition into single parenthood had a significantly higher rate of depression than their married counterparts at 'Time 1,' which increased, but not significantly, at 'Time 2' (Wade & Cairney, 2000). Data for this study was collected from longitudinal National Population Health Surveys (NPHS) by Statistics Canada in 1994 and in 1996. The subjects consisted of 2169 women between the ages of 20 and 65 years with children living at home. Reasons for separation for the single mothers included lack of affection and of commitment on the part of their partners, and more arguments.

The findings were similar to the previous study to the extent that, compared to their married counterparts, mothers transiting into single parenthood had a significantly higher rate of major depression at Time 1, which increased, though not significantly, by Time 2. Making a transition into a marital relationship did not decrease their depression to any significant degree from stable single mother at Time 1 or Time 2. Movement into marriage did not seem to serve any protective function. Rates of depression among married and single mothers tended to be quite stable, with single mothers twice as likely to experience a major episode of depression in the preceding twelve months. Adequate income did partially mediate depression, but social support had no mediating effect.

The next study, however, found that inadequate social support explained to a significant degree the presence of depression in single parents in a population-based investigation (Cairney, Boyle, Offord, & Racine, 2003). A secondary data analysis of the 1994–5 National Population Health Survey yielded a total of 2921 subjects, of whom 17,626 single and married mothers participated in this study. Through a process of exclusion and elimination, the final sample consisted of 725 single mothers and 2231 married mothers.

Results showed that over a period of twelve months, single mothers were more susceptible to have suffered an episode of depression than their married counterparts. They also reported higher levels of chronic stress, more recent life-events, more childhood adversities, and more problems with their children. Single mothers also experienced lower levels of social support and social interaction with friends and family than did married mothers. Stress and social support combined accounted for 40% of the relationship between single-parent status and depression. One overarching conclusion of this study was that social stressors had the most impact in terms of accounting for a relationship between single-parent status and depression.

Given the relatively common presence of depression in single mothers, are they likely to make greater demands on mental health services? Cairney and Wade (2002) examined that question by employing a secondary analysis of the 1994–5 National Population Health Survey. The study sample consisted of 512 single mothers and 2549 married mothers between the ages of 15 and 54. Some of the key findings were that single mothers with the diagnosis of a major depressive episode were significantly more likely to utilize mental health services than married mothers with the same condition. The same differences in the utilization of mental health services emerged between single mothers and married mothers who did not meet the criteria of a major depressive episode. Single-parent status alone was found to be a major predictor of metal-health-services utilization that was independent of depression. Overall, single mothers were more likely to have sought professional help and had a higher rate of mental-health-service use than married mothers. Just being single mothers increased their risk for poor mental health, resulting in a higher use of mental health services.

Our final study in this section examines several factors that would seem to be associated with major depression in mothers, including lone mothers (Lara-Cinisomo & Griffin, 2007). The subjects in this study were drawn in 2000–1 from Wave 1 of the Los Angeles Family and Neighborhood Survey, derived from 65 census tracts. Altogether 1865 ethnically mixed subjects participated in this study. The largest group was Hispanic (62%) followed by white/non- Hispanic (21%), Black (8%), and Asian (8%). They included married (64%), cohabiting (12%), and single mothers (24%). Altogether 15% of the total sample was depressed. Depression was more common in single mothers (19%) than either married (12%) or cohabiting (16%). Single mothers had significantly higher odds of having major depression compared with married mothers. Mothers with a college degree or beyond (17%) were significantly less likely to be depressed than mothers without a college degree (83%). Finally, mothers with only adolescent children were significantly more likely to have a major depression than mothers without. The fact of being a single mother alone may not be the best predictor of depression. However, if the single mother does not posses a college education and has one or more adolescent children at home, the risk for depression is likely to be very high.

Summary

Single parenthood is fraught with challenges. Poverty, an elevated risk of morbidity, and even mortality and social isolation may be only a partial list of the many woes confronting single mothers. Even children growing up with a single mother may confront many more obstacles than children with two parents. One question that is not adequately addressed in the body of research on single parenthood is the degree to which poverty may be responsible for much of the parents' problems. It is not altogether surprising that depression appears to be endemic to single motherhood. Brown and Moran (1997) made an important observation, suggesting that it would be simplistic to invoke poverty as the root cause of depression and other problems in single mothers. Social isolation, the burdens of child-rearing, and the effort that it took to work full time also conspired to predispose these women to depression. And yet, the irrefutable fact is that in Canada single mothers continue to be among the poorest. The relationship between poverty and depression is beyond question. Brown and Harris (1978) alerted us to the likelihood of social factors being of major etiologic significance in the causation of depression in women. That sad fact seems as prevalent now, especially in the context of single mothers, as it was over three decades ago.

Does Marriage/Long-Term Relationship Promote Health?

The life-event and social-support literature provides ample evidence for the power of an intimate and reciprocal relationship to mitigate, or even ameliorate, the ill effects of negative life-events. Here, we seek evidence that goes beyond the life-event research, and examine the broader population-based studies to seek support or its lack for this proposition.

It must be acknowledged at the outset that there is truly an abundance of scientific literature on this topic. We have endeavoured to focus on a few population-based studies. Nevertheless, despite this shortcoming, we hope that our conclusions reflect the key research findings on this critical subject. The subject is critical because of the changing nature of families and a significant rise in single-person households. Does being single, by definition, increases the health risk or, obversely, does being married or in a long-term relationship predict better health.

In the section preceding we discussed the down side of single parent-hood. In recent literature the status of the single person (not necessarily a single parent) has received considerable scrutiny. In a review of the data on marital status and mortality due to neoplasms and cardiovas-cular diseases in Canada between 1951 and 1981, Trovato and Lauris (1989) concluded that married persons had a lower death rate than the unmarried. A transition from married to unmarried generally favoured men more than it favoured women. Men shared a greater reduction in mortality from a change in marital status (from unmarried to married).

The authors offered a number of possibilities that may account for these findings: (1) married persons have higher socio-economic sta-tus than the unmarried; (2) life expectancy could be linked to a stress factor inherent in the change of a marital status, positive for marriage and negative for widowhood or divorce; (3) marriage may be selective for healthier persons; and (4) marriage may have a socially integrative functions. Some of these observations are challenged by other research findings presently discussed.

DePaulo and Morris (2005), in a sweeping review of this topic, argued that single-hood, far from being of high risk for morbidity and mortality (as our review will show), is a product of the ideology of marriage and family. We only present some of their key observations.

They begin by pointing out that in 2002 there were 86 million single adults in the United States. Another fact of import they emphasize is that Americans now spend more of their adult life single than married. The only fact that separates single from married is the absence of a sexual partner. These authors point out that this particular gap is often offset by the presence of close and enduring friendships. And not having a sexual partner does not necessarily translate into not having sex. The research also feeds into supporting the stigmatization of singles. The authors argue their case from the following perspectives: evolutionary psychology, attachment theory, a social problems standpoint, the growth of the cult of the couple, and the appeal of an ideology that offers a simple and compelling world view.

We consider this article important for two reasons: (1) the predominance of research that affirms the value of a lasting relationship, and (2) the need for a new approach to research incorporating the ideas discussed in the article. Byrne and Carr (2005), responding to the article, made these points: first, that single persons do not experience institutional discrimination; second, never-married persons were likely to face discrimination in informal relationships and interpersonal exchanges. Compared to men, never-married women were more likely to report that they were treated with less respect. While being single may increase certain kinds of health risks, long-term low-quality marriage has the capacity to have significant effects on overall well-being (Hawkins & Booth, 2005).

In a longitudinal study (Hawkins & Booth, 2005), the negative fallout from low-quality marriage was explored. This study utilized the first four waves of the Marital Instability Over the Life-Course Study. The sample consisted of 2033 married individuals under the age of 55 who were living with their spouses. A number of hypotheses were put to the test. The most critical and perhaps predictable finding was that people in low-quality marriage experience many negative effects on their overall well-being. Among the more pronounced consequences were elevated levels of psychological distress compared to the remaining-continually-married couples in the sample, lowered life-satisfaction, lower self-esteem, and significantly lower levels of overall happiness. There was some evidence which showed that staying unhappily married was more detrimental than divorcing.

The fact that troubled marriages can be harmful to health was supported in a comprehensive review of the literature on the consequences of marriage (Robles & Keicolt-Glaser, 1989). Marital quality has been shown to have measurable impact on cardiovascular, endocrine, and immune functions. The exhaustive review led to the following conclusions: (1) The evidence from marital-interaction studies point in the direction that marital strain could produce negative consequences for cardiovascular, endocrine, and immune functions. There may even be long-term negative effects as well as difficulties in recovering from a wound and susceptibility to infections. Second, the investigations on marital interactions and physiological pathways were generally conducted with relatively healthy couples, thus limiting the generalizability of the research findings. Third, there exists a dearth of data on the relationship between marital interaction and physiology and health outcomes. More research utilizing experimental designs would provide greater and more precise control over specific aspects of marital interaction that may be important to isolate.

Our next report examines the question of gender in marriage (Williams, 2003). Do women and men respond differentially to different attributes of marriage? Data was derived from a nationally representative sample of 3617 persons over the age of 24 and older residing in the continental United States. The original sample was interviewed in 1986, and subsequently 65% of that number (n=2348) in 1989 and 1994. The measures included marital status continuity and change, marital quality, psychological well-being, and socio-demographic control variables.

The following were the key findings: The data failed to support the hypothesis that marriage provides greater psychological benefits to men than women. Second, the transition into a second marriage is associated with a decline in depression and an increase in life-satisfaction for men only. Third, the results failed to support the proposition that the quality of the marital relationship was more important to women's psychological well-being than to men's; high levels of marital stress and low levels of marital harmony were equally responsible for undermining life-satisfaction for both women and men. Fourth, the results for depression and life-satisfaction indicated that for men and women it was better to be continually unmarried that to be in an even moderately unsatisfying marriage. Fifth, when the Time 1 quality of marriage was poor, those who went through divorce, separation, or widowhood did not report significantly greater increases in depression than the continually married. Only when life-satisfaction was high on Time 1, did leaving marriage increase depression. Among women with Time 1 poor-quality marriage, a transition to widowhood was associated with increased life-satisfaction.

The overall conclusion was that, with few exceptions, the effects of marital stress, marital transitions, and marital quality on psychological well-being were similar for men and women. Besides, in some circumstances, being single increased life-satisfaction. The authors concluded that not much was known about the process of remarriage and its influence on men's and women's mental health. Much more research was called for to fully appreciate this particular transition for both genders.

The next study (Liu & Umberson, 2008) furnished at least partial support for the preceding one. The premise of this study was that while significant changes had occurred both in the meaning and rates of being married, separated, never-married, and widowed over the past many decades, there is little knowledge about the historical trends in the relationship between marital status and health. To this end the authors used repeated cross-sectional data from the National Health Interview Survey from 1972 to 2003 to analyse historical trends in marital-status differentials in health. We report their findings in broad terms.

The results indicated that, over the period studied, the probability of reporting good health increased modestly among the married, but it increased at a much faster pace among the never-married, thus the gap between the two groups was narrowing over time. However, the probability of reporting good health declined among the divorced, separated, and especially the widowed. This widened the gap between the married and the rest over the 1970–2003 period. Level of income had little impact on health status among the various groups.

Gender, however, emerged as a significant factor. The gap between the married and the never-married has converged over time for men, but not for women. Furthermore, the adverse effects of divorce were more pronounced for women than men. The authors concluded that their findings raised serious issues about some long-held beliefs. They emphasized three gender-related changes: First, their findings suggested that while the health of married men remained stable over the time span, women's self-reported health, in fact, improved. Second, the apparent advantage for the married over the never-married remained stable over time for women, but diminished for men. Third, the increasing gap between the married and previously married in self-reports of health was even more pronounced for women than men. Their findings may have major social significance in that the self-reported health for never-married men was increasingly similar to that of married men over time. The seeming health advantage of being married was diminished over time in relation to the never-married. However, being married was still advantageous in relation to the health of the widowed, divorced, and separated, especially for women. Losing a partner as opposed to never having one seems to produce different health effects.

Finally, we report, albeit briefly, an investigation on the effects of social support on mortality among seniors (Wilkins, 2003). This analysis was based on longitudinal household data from the National Population Health Survey for 2422 persons aged 65 and over in 1994–5. A truly astonishing finding was that married men experienced 40% less risk of death than their non-married counterparts. Participation in organizations also reduced the risk of death. As for gender differences, a clear relationship emerged between social support and mortality for men, but no such association was found for women. The author cautioned that this sex difference was not caused by insufficient statistical power. Rather, this may be a fundamental difference. An example of this difference may be attributed to women perhaps being more vulnerable than men to the negative aspect of social relations. In addition, they are more likely to assume a caretaking role. This is an important paper for providing information on the relationship between social support and mortality in seniors.

Summary

The literature on marriage and its relationship to health literature produced very complex results. Being single may not be as perilous as we might imagine. There indeed is no linear relationship between being married and enjoying better health. The gender differences are intriguing in this equation. Quality of marriage is equally important. In some instances, divorce is a better alternative to staying in a low-quality marriage. Marriage may prolong life, but men shared a greater reduction in mortality from changing status from unmarried to married. On the other hand, the effects of marital stress, marital transition, and marital quality on psychological well-being was similar for both sexes. Marriage may be good for better health, but it comes with many conditions.

Conclusion

Research, in broad terms, confirms the role of the intimate and reciprocal partner relationship as a major source of social support with many positive attributes. However, as we attempted to show, over the past three decades the very idea of marriage and family has undergone almost a revolutionary change. The sheer rise in the number of single-person households attests to that. Single parenthood in Canada and elsewhere has almost become synonymous with poverty and other social disadvantages. And yet, we have new forms of single parenthood that did not exist thirty or forty years ago. An example of this would be a highly educated single woman choosing to have a baby. There are more variations on the definition of family than ever before.

In the final section of this chapter we explored the benefits and fallout of marriage by focusing on population-based studies. Being single, in itself, need not be a disadvantage. More research is required to further our understanding. Gender and quality of marriage are key determinants of the social support aspect of the marriage relationship. Thus, while marriage, on the whole, promotes health as well longevity, it come with many provisions.

REFERENCES

BBC Online Health (2001). Britain becomes a nation of loners. 11 December.

Brown, G., & Harris, T. (1978). *Social origins of depression: A study of psychiatric disorders in women*. London: Tavistock Publications Ltd.

Brown, G., & Moran, P. (1997). Single mothers, poverty and depression. *Psychological Medicine, 27*, 21–33.

Byrne, A., & Carr, D. (2005). Commentaries. Caught in the cultural lag: The stigma of singlehood. *Psychological Inquiry, 16*: 85–97.

Cairney, J., Boyle, M., Offord, D., & Racine, Y. (2003). Stress, social support and depression in single and married mothers. *Social Psychiatry & Psychiatric Epidemiology, 38*, 442–449.

Cairney, J., & Wade, T. (2002). Single parent mothers and mental health care service use. *Social Psychiatry and Psychiatric Epidemiology, 37*, 236–242.

CBC Television. *DOC ZONE*. 'Bio-Dad.' 26 February 2009 (broadcast date).

Cohen, S., & Wills, T. (1985). Stress, social support, and the buffering hypothesis. *Psychological Bulletin, 98*: 310–357.

Coyne, J., & DeLongis, A. (1986). Going beyond social support: The role of social relationships in adaptation. *Journal of Consulting and Clinical Psychology, 54*, 454 460.

Curtis, L., & Phipps, S. (2004). Social transfers and the health of single mothers in Norway and Canada. *Social Sc. Medicine, 58*, 2499–2557.

DePaulo, B., & Morris, W. (2005). Singles in society and science. *Psychological Inquiry, 16*, 57–83.

Guttmann, A., Dick, P., & To, T. (2004). Infant hospitalization and maternal depression, poverty and single parenthood – A population-based study. *Child: Care, Health and Development, 30*, 60–75.

Harris, M., Greco, P., Wysocki, T., Elder-Danda, C., & White, N. (1999). Adolescents with diabetes from single-parent, blended, and in-tact families: Health related and family functioning. *Families, Systems, and Health, 17*: 181–196.

Harrison, J., Maguire, P., & Pitceathly, C. (1995). Confiding in crisis: Gender differences in patterns of confiding among cancer patients. *Social Science and Medicine, 41*, 1255 1260.

Hawkins, D., & Booth, A. (2005). Unhappily ever after: Effects of long-term, low-quality marriages on well-being. *Social Forces, 84*, 451–468.

Lara-Cinisomo, S., & Griffin, B. (2007). Factors associated with major depression among mothers in Los Angeles. *Women's Health Issues, 17*, 316–324.

Liu, H., & Umberson, D. (2008). The times they are a changin': Marital status and health differentials from 1972 to 2003. *J. Health & Social Behavior, 49*, 239–253.

Lorant, V., Croux, C., Weich, S., Deliege, D., et al. (2007). Depression and socioeconomic risk factor: 7 year longitudinal population study. *Br. J. Psychiatry, 190*, 293–298.

Manne, S., Ostroff, J., Winkel, G., Grana, G., & Fox, K. (2005). Partner unsupportive responses, avoidant coping, and distress among women with early stage breast cancer: Patient and partner perspectives. *Health Psychology, 24*, 635–641.

McCashin, A. (1996). *Lone mothers in Ireland: A local study*. Dublin: Oak Tree Press.

McFarlane, A., Norman, G., Streiner, D., & Roy, R. (1983). The process of social stress: Stable, reciprocal, and mediating relationships. *J. Health & Social Behavior, 24*, 160–173.

Neises, G., & Gruneberg, C. (2005). Socioeconomic situation and health outcomes of single parents. *J. Public Health, 13*, 270–278.

Penninx, B., van Tilburg, T., Boeke, A., Deeg, D., et al. (1998). Effects of social support and personal coping resources on depressive symptoms: Different for various chronic diseases? *Health Psychology, 17*, 551–558.

Ringback, W., Haglund, B., & Rosen, M. (2000). Mortality among lone mothers in Sweden: A population study. *Lancet, 355,* 1215–1259.

Robles, T., & Kiecolt-Glaser, J. (1989). The physiology of marriage: Pathways to health. *J. Marriage and Family, 51,* 907–922.

Sauvola, A., Rasanen, P., Joukamaa, M., Jokelainen, J., et al. (2001). Mortality of young adults in relation to single-parent family background. *European J. Public Health, 11,* 284–286.

Sherman, J., & DeVinney, D. (2004). Social support and adjustment after spinal cord injury: Influence of past peer-mentoring experiences and current live-in partner. *Rehabilitation Psychol., 49,* 140–149.

Statistics Canada (2006a). *Family portrait: Continuity and change in Canadian families and households in 2006.* National portrait: Households. Ottawa, Canada.

Statistics Canada (2006b) *Family portrait: Continuity and change in Canadian families and households in 2006.* National portrait: Census families. Ottawa, Canada.

Thoits, P. (1995). Stress, coping and social support processes: Where are we? What next? *J. Health & Social Behavior, 35,* 53–79.

Trovato, F., & Lauris, G. (1989). Marital status and mortality in Canada: 1951–1981. *J. Marriage and the Family, 51,* 907–922.

Wade, T., & Cairney, J. (2000). Major depressive disorder and marital transition among mothers: Results from a National Panel Study. *J. Mental & Nervous Disease, 188,* 741–750.

Walker, A., Maher, J., Coulthard, M., Goddard, W., & Thomas, M. (2000–1). *Living in Britain: Results from 2000–2001 General Household Survey.* London, HMSO.

Whitehead, M., Burstrom, B., & Diderichsen, F. (2000). Social policies and pathways to inequalities in health: A comparative analysis of lone mothers in Britain and Sweden. *Social Science & Medicine, 50,* 255–270.

Wilkins, K. (2003). Social support and mortality in seniors. *Health Reports, 14,* 21–34.

Williams, K. (2003). Has the future of marriage arrived? A contemporary examination of gender, marriage, and psychological well-being. *J. Health and Social Behavior, 44,* 470–487.

4 Chronic Pain and Social Support

Pain is defined by the International Association for the Study of Pain (IASP) as 'an unpleasant sensory and emotional experience associated with actual or potential tissue damage, or described in terms of such damage.' Chronic pain, in addition to these characteristics, is usually of three or more months' duration, or longer, and is generally unresponsive to conventional medical interventions. Chronic pain is widespread. In the United States 40% of the adult population is affected by chronic pain. Estimates in terms of its social cost (medical expense, lost income, lost productivity) are well over $100 billion annually (*Pain Medicine*, 2005). In Canada, according to National Population Health Survey, 1994–5, some 20% women and 15% men suffer from some form of chronic pain.

The psychological and social effects of chronic pain are also substantial (Roy, 2007; Tunks, Crook, & Weir, 2008; Tunks, Weir, & Crook, 2008). In their exhaustive review, the latter researchers noted the presence of psychological co-morbidity, which added a high degree of complication to chronic pain that could have a significant impact on prognosis. Depression was ubiquitous in this population. In addition, abuse, employment handicaps, poor coping skills, and other social factors were commonly found (Tunks, Weir, & Crook, 2008). They concluded that the weight of epidemiologic evidence made it clear that chronic pain was best understood in the context of the psychosocial environment.

In a cross-sectional study with a postal survey to 3928 subjects of the adult general population, followed by clinical examination of subjects with no pain, chronic regional pain, chronic widespread pain, chronic widespread pain (Manchester definition), and fibromyalgia, Bergman (2005) reported that the latter three groups were found to present with more severe impairment of health than the other two groups. Psycho social factors such as lower socio-economic status, being an immigrant, compromised housing, a lower educational level, combined with lower social support, explained the higher level of pain in the chronic wide-spread pain and fibromyalgia subjects, but not so with the no-pain and regional pain subjects.

Roy (2007) noted that major disruptions in the social environment of a chronic pain sufferer were predictable. Job loss, disruption in family rules and roles, sometimes a massive shrinking of the social support network, and higher dependence on the medical and other formal systems were commonly noted. Psychosocial issues along with psychological complications are endemic to chronic pain. Inadequate social support is far from uncommon. In the rest of this chapter we investigate the question of social support by examining (1) the broad literature on social support and chronic pain with an emphasis on chronic low-back pain (CLBP) and fibromyalgia (two conditions common among the pain clinic population, and (2) the spouse as a source of social support (a well-researched area with chronic pain patients).

Social Support and Chronic Pain

Given the magnitude of social disruption that seems to accompany chronic pain, it is not at all surprising that social support is one of the not-so-infrequent casualties. There is now over two decades of research on the value of social support in coping with chronic pain (Roy 2001). Roy's review concluded that the weight of the literature did find support for the buffering hypothesis of social support for chronic pain. However, in his review of social support and rheumatoid arthritis (RA), he concluded that the research outcome was inconclusive. Only a handful of studies examined the effects of buffering on the overall functioning of patients with RA. Some studies did find a buffering effect, and others found either a weak effect or none. In relation to headache, he noted that the studies lacked a central theme, and there seemed to be a focus on the consequences of a lack of social support rather any attempt to test the buffering hypothesis. The chronic low-back pain and social support literature also produced complex results. They were extraordinarily varied in scope and methodology, which made drawing any general conclusion a daring undertaking. Below we discuss a sample of recent studies involving general chronic pain patients and the buffering hypothesis.

To begin with, we discuss three recent papers that addressed the question of perceived social support and their role in (1) pain-related catastrophizing (Buenaver, Edwards, & Haythornthwaite, 2007); (2) pain adjustment (Lopez-Martinez, Esteve Zarazaga, & Ramirez-Maestre, 2008), and (3) coping with fatigue in patients suffering from Systemic Lupus Erythematosus (SLE) (Jump et al., 2005).

In a sample of 1356 patients, Buenaver and associates tested whether association between catastrophizing and negative pain-related outcomes was influenced by patients' perceptions of significant others' responses to their pain. Catastrophizing is a not infrequent phenomenon among chronic pain sufferers. It implies magnification, associated with helplessness and pessimism. Chronic pain patients are often without an adequate explanation for their pain, which can be debilitating. Under such circumstances, it may not be unusual for patients to harbour fear of the unknown. Depression is a known contributory factor for catastrophizing.

Some of the key findings were: (1) catastrophizing was strongly associated with perceived punishing responses among patients perceiving lower social support; (2) a low level of perceived social support was associated with pain-related disability; (3) perceived social responses were found to have a marginal effect in mediating the relationship between catastrophizing and pain-related outcomes; and (4) these effects were not observed among patients with higher social support. The authors noted several limitations of this study, among them the cross-sectional design, which precluded any causal associations and, very critically, the fact that subjects' pain conditions were undiagnosed. As such, the findings demand cautious interpretation. Nonetheless, perceived rather than actual and measurable social support is a factor that needs to be taken into account in any assessment of the chronic-pain patients' environment.

A Spanish study (Lopez-Martinez, Esteve-Zarazaga, & Ramirez-Maestre, 2008) tested a hypothetical model of the associations between perceived social support, coping responses to pain, pain intensity, functional disability, and a depressed mood. The subjects for this study were recruited from a pain clinic population; 117 patients agreed to participate. Valid instruments were used for data collection. The findings were unequivocal to the degree that there was a strong relationship between perceived social support and a depressed mood and pain intensity, but not with functional disability. These results showed that higher levels of perceived social support generally result in less passive pain coping strategies. These results contradicted earlier findings that perceived social support led to a more adaptive pain coping proving beneficial for a long-term outcome. The authors noted several short-comings in this study, most notably the use of self-report measures and a cross-sectional study design, which meant that no causal relationship could be invoked.

Our final paper in this section (Jump et al., 2005) reported on an investigation of the buffering effect of perceived social support in dealing with fatigue in patients with SLE. The participants were 127 patients with SLE. The mean age of the patients was 40.6 years and the duration of illness ranged from one to 38 years. Standardized measures were used to measure pain, fatigue, severity of pain, and depression.

The results showed a moderate association between fatigue and pain intensity. Fatigue in this study emerged as an important feature of SLE, and it was the most highly rated symptom compared to other complaints. Fatigue scores were significantly higher than all other assessed symptoms. However, neither fatigue nor pain intensity were significantly related to disease activity. Perceived social support was inversely correlated with depression as well as fatigue. The buffering function of perceived social support received confirmation in this study.

Summary

Our review of the role of perceived social support as a buffer against chronic pain produced a mixed outcome. In dealing with catastrophizing pain, as we noted, the results were complex, and yet subjects with higher social support did not show the same effects as those with lower perceived support. With the mixed-chronic-pain (undiagnosed) population, the value of perceived social support was significantly associated with a depressed mood and pain intensity. With SLE, the buffering role of perceived social support was confirmed. Worthy of attention is an earlier study which tested the buffering hypothesis in mitigating negative mood and the effects on pain in a group of patients with reflex sympathetic dystrophy syndrome (Feldman & Downey, 1999). Perceived social support had both main and buffering effects on negative mood, and a main effect on pain. In essence, perceived social support is a positive force in mitigating in varying degrees the ill effects of chronic pain disorders in diverse populations. Differences in outcome, at least in part, can be explained by methodological differences, shortcomings such as reliance on patient self-report, and diverse populations.

Population-Based Studies

Population-based studies related to social support and chronic pain are few and far between. We present two rather diverse studies, one of which compares rural versus urban populations (Hoffman, Meier, & Council, 2002), and the second, Caucasians versus African American (Ruehlman, Karoly, & Newton, 2008) chronic-pain populations and the effects of social support.

Hoffman and associates conducted a population-based study with the following objectives: (1) to establish the overall prevalence and reported experience of chronic pain in North Dakota; (2) to compare the characteristics of chronic pain across rural and urban populations; (3) to evaluate the impact of chronic pain on quality of life; and (4) to explore the effects of social support on chronic pain.

Their sample was drawn from a survey of 1550 North Dakota residents. A total of 188 inhabitants responded to the mail survey, and eventually 96 rural subjects and 92 urban subjects completed the study. Chronic pain was defined as a constant pain or pain that flared up often and had persisted for six months at a time. Social support was measured using the Social Constrained Scale, which is designed to elicit information about sharing one's feelings freely with others.

Sixty-three out of 96 rural subjects (65.6%) and 46 out of 92 urban subjects (50%) met the criteria of pain. More rural than urban subjects reported chronic pain. For both rural and urban subjects, significant relationships emerged between intensity of chronic pain and the number of treatments received, quality of life and the self-reported adequacy of health care, and the intensity and duration of chronic pain.

The results in relation to social support were complex, and the notion that a larger family support network would lower the social constraints in discussing chronic pain with others was not supported. Authors noted that as the size of rural households increased, individuals felt less able to discuss freely their pain-related concerns. The size of the support system was not a mitigating factor. However, better quality of life and lower social constraints (social support) were evident in the entire rural sample. This, however, was not true for the urban sample, which showed that quality of life and social constraints were not significantly related. There was general support for the hypothesis that support from family and friends was helpful in coping with pain. However, there was an absence of such a relationship between quality of life and social constraints.

A critical question that this survey failed to explain was, if social support helped in coping more effectively with pain, why did it fail to improve the overall quality of life. This study had many methodological shortcomings. Its measure for social support did not adequately assess either its quality or the buffering effects. The instrument used (Social Constraints Scale) is, at best, an indirect measure of social support, measuring people's ability to communicate their negative emotions about painful subjects. It does not address one of the key components of social support, which is reciprocity. Another key omission is the absence of any information about the presence of key persons in the support system rather than its size. In broad terms, the survey did show the benefits related to some aspects of social support in coping with pain for both rural and urban pain sufferers. It would be an error to draw too many conclusions from this study.

In an examination of the psychosocial dimensions of chronic pain in Caucasians and African Americans (Ruehlman, Karoly, & Newton, 2008), the authors explored the experience of social support between the two groups. The African American subjects were drawn from a national sample of 2407 participants, which contained a total of 214 non-Hispanic African Americans. The 214 Caucasian subjects were randomly selected from a set of 1934.

The experience of pain was remarkably similar between the two groups. No significant differences emerged in pain severity, interference, emotional burden, or treatment status. However, it was noteworthy that African Americans relied more heavily than their Caucasian counterparts on off-the-counter medicine for pain control. Significant differences emerged between the two groups on psychosocial variables. African American subjects were found to be more vulnerable in the domain of beliefs. They entertained many counter-productive beliefs and attitudes.

The picture that emerged for social support was mixed. While the African American subjects were more likely to identify and confide in someone significant in their network and also reported significantly higher emotional support than their white counterparts, this was counteracted by many negative social responses and insensitivity, probably undoing the benefits of social support.

The authors noted that the role of social negativity has often been overlooked in favour of social support in the literature. And yet social support and social negativity have both been linked to important outcomes among chronic pain sufferers. The most critical fact to emerge from this study was that African Americans were more likely than Caucasians to identify the most important person as the provider of social support. However, the same individual also demonstrated impatience and insensitivity. The net effect of such behaviour, in the end, may be to undermine the patient's effort to adapt.

Summary

The last two studies, both using survey design, varied significantly in their methodology and execution. The urban-rural study (Hoffman, Meier, & Council, 2002) had many limitations, with rather scanty information on social support. The Ruehlman and associates study (2008), by contrast, was complex and identified an interesting aspect of social support not often addressed in the pain–social support literature, namely, the source of major support also acting as the major critic, thus undoing the positive aspects of support. We may be able to address that issue presently as we examine spousal social support as a help or hindrance. First, however, social support is examined in relation to (1) chronic low-back pain and (2) fibromyalgia.

Social Support and Chronic Low-Back Pain

Social support research in relation to chronic low-back pain (CLBP) is diverse and does not lend itself to meaningful categorization. The literature ranges from the role of social factors, among other psychosocial variables, in predicting chronicity and quality of life in patients with CLBP (Koleck et al., 2006) to the effects of negative partner response in CLBP patients in their satisfaction with relationships (Waxman, Tripp, & Flamenbaum, 2008). An earlier study (Turner, Clancy, and Vitaliano, 1987) showed the beneficial effect of seeking social support as it was negatively related to present-pain rating on the McGill Pain Questionnaire. An Israeli study (Reis, Hermoni, Borkan, et al., 1999) found the strongest predictors of chronicity in patients with a history of low-back pain were depression, job changes due to back pain, family delegitimization of pain, lack of social support, coping style, and unemployment among other factors. Another study also found support for low social support as a predictor of low-back pain chronicity in Navy servicemen (Patel, 2007). Taken together, all these studies confirm the positive role of social support in moderating pain or better adjustment or in avoiding chronicity. Below we discuss two major papers in some depth to show the buffering power of social support in relation to low-back pain in non-clinical populations in their work environment.

In a sweeping review of the literature on the relationship between work-related musculoskeletal pain and social support, Woods (2005) concluded that there existed good evidence to support an association between poor social support and an increased risk for musculoskeletal morbidity. This review was based on 52 studies, most of which were conducted in Scandinavia, followed by the United States, Canada, and Europe. It is noteworthy that the results from methodologically weaker studies were included because they produced richly detailed information. The overall results from a review of cross-sectional, case control, as well as prospective quantitative and qualitative studies, showed that there was powerful evidence for an association between poor social support at work and musculoskeletal morbidity. The lack of support at work experienced by the workers was generally from their co-workers, supervisors, or managers. This review is of considerable significance, as it goes well beyond the established concerns about the relationship between intimate social support and health. The power of social support extends well beyond the circle of friends and relations.

Eriksen and associates (2004) conducted a major study on work factors that predicted CLBP in nurses' aides. The authors randomly selected 12,000 nurses aides from the union members' list, and mailed them a questionnaire. After one reminder, 7478 consented to participate and completed the questionnaire. Out of that group, 4266 met the inclusion criteria, and with the dropouts, the final number of participants was 3808. In addition to demographic data, information related to work performance and psychological and social factors that included social support at work, fairness of the immediate superior's leadership, and rewards for good work was obtained.

At the three-month follow-up, 14.1% reported being intensely bothered by LBP during the previous three months, while another 4% reported one or several LBP-related sick leaves lasting longer than three days. At the fifteen-month follow-up, 6.3% reported one or more LBP-related sick leaves lasting longer than 14 days in the previous 12 months.

The results revealed that 'a culture in the work unit that was perceived as "some," "rather much," or "very much" supportive or encouraging was associated with lower odds of LBP related sick leaves exceeding three days than a culture that was perceived as "not at all, very little or rather little" supportive or encouraging' (p. 401). Among other factors, during the fifteen-month observation period, reduced perceived support and encouragement predicted LBP-related sick days exceeding 14 days.

The authors were careful to point out that in a cross-sectional study of Swedish nurses (Ahlberg-Hulten, Theorell, & Sigala, 1995), no association between social support and LBP was found. Another study (Logerstrom et al., 1995), however, found an association between low social support at work and low-back symptoms (not severe) in a group of hospital nurses in Sweden. The Eriksen study, however, found powerful evidence of a relationship between perceived lack of support from the immediate superior and intense LBP.

Summary

There is general support for the proposition that social support does play a part in mitigating chronic low-back pain and that intimates and family members are central sources for this support. Yet, the major review along with the study of nursing aides add an important perspective, namely, situation-specific social support. Support in the workplace from peers and immediate supervisors emerged as exerting varying degrees of buffering effect on the overall well-being of the workers, and the absence of such support caused low-back pain. Poor social support also seemed to be associated with higher levels of morbidity with CLBP.

Headache and Social Support

Headaches are a common medical affliction experienced by a large segment of the population. They can range from very transient to severe and debilitating. The ailment is a collection of disorders, and is classified into many discreet conditions. In this section we review four studies, first, to develop an appreciation of the role of social support and its buffering function and, second, to consider the sheer scope of the research studies related to social support and headaches.

Our first, earlier, study is a three-stage study of stress related to life-events and headache and social support (Martin & Theunissen, 1993) Subjects for this study were recruited through a newspaper advertisement. Inclusion criteria included (a) an average headache frequency of a minimum of once a week; (b) a duration of at least twelve months; (c) a medical diagnosis of migraine and tension-type headache; and (d) an age range of 19–59 years. Twenty-eight headache subjects completed the study. Standardized instruments were used to measure life-events and social support. Four distinct aspects of social support were included: (1) availability of attachment; (2) adequacy of attachment; (3) availability of social integration; and (4) adequacy of social integration.

Study 1 found that the chronic headache sufferers did not differ from non-headache controls in terms of stress from life-events or coping skills. They did, however, differ in one critical dimension of social support, namely, the availability of social integration. Study 2, with a different control group, found further support for all four types of social support for the patient population compared to the controls. The third study was not directly relevant to our purposes.

The results failed to find any significant differences between the two types of headache sufferers, in terms of either life-events or coping skills, which included social support. The authors noted that the results found clear support for a difference between chronic headache sufferers and the somewhat different non-headache control groups in Studies 1 and 2.

This study proposed that low social support made individuals vulnerable to headaches via a stress-buffering effect or that low social support meant a higher stress level. The data supported this proposition. The authors also proposed that an alternative view of the findings was that chronic headaches could also lead to low social support as they might create difficulties in maintaining social relationships. Further research was called for to understand the aspects of social support that were deficient in headache sufferers, and to unravel the directions of causality.

A comprehensive Dutch study (Vos & Passchier, 2003) investigated the factors that might account for a reduced impact of migraine on the lives of these patients. Migraine impacts on virtually every aspect of life – physical, psychological, and social. Subjects for this study were recruited from the Dutch Society of Headache Patients. Altogether, 448 members responded to a set of standard and structured questionnaires which included the Migraine-Specific Quality of Life Instrument (MSQOL). Some 70% of this group reported a number of factors that had made migraines more tolerable or reduced their impact.

Results were telling. Patients benefited from support from a variety of sources that helped them to reduce the negative consequences of this disease. A majority of patients (70%) experienced improvement in their disease just with medication, which was not altogether unpredictable. Other factors that had a mitigating effect on the disease were lifestyle change, more relaxed coping with the disease, leading a more regular life, and managing stress at work. The direct benefit of social support was frequently mentioned, which included the Dutch Society of Headache Patients (58%), family (46%), and the patients' general practitioners (28%). Patients who reported less impact had fewer migraine attacks and enjoyed a higher quality of life than those who failed to report such a reduction.

This large-scale clinical-population-based study demonstrated the wide range of sources of social support. While there is recognition of the value of intimate relationship for having a buffering function or even for preventing morbidity, this study revealed that problem-specific support such as that from family physicians or peers, in addition to family, could be very effective.

The next study (Peters, Abu-Sadd, Robbins, Vydelingum, et al., 2005) examined the following strategies used by migraine and chronic daily headache patients: (1) health care consultations; (2) medication and alternative remedies; (3) acute and prophylactic strategies; and (4) social support. Three groups, namely, patients with migraine, migraine with aura, and chronic daily headaches, were compared. A postal questionnaire was sent to 887 members of the Migraine Action Association, UK. Four hundred and thirty-eight questionnaires were analysed. The three groups of patients did not significantly differ in age, gender, ethnicity, level of education, or employment status. Significant differences emerged in the way the three groups used headache specialists, neurologists, acute medications, antidepressants, and some acute and prophylactic avoidance techniques. No significant differences emerged between the groups in their use of other health professionals and alternative health professionals, general acute management, or use of social support. Yet, these strategies were actively used.

One key finding of direct relevance to this chapter was the limited use of social support by the three groups of patients. This was indeed the least used of all strategies. Social support came from three sources: (1) the media, (2) family and friends, and (3) other headache patients (peer support). Support groups and helplines were used by more than 30% of the respondents. The authors did not offer any explanation for this finding. This study did establish that use of social support was part of a coping repertoire for a significant proportion of chronic headache sufferers. No data related to the differences, if any, between users and non-users of social support was provided. Nor was any explanation offered for such limited use of social support by the three groups of patients.

Our final study (Skomo, Desselle, & Berdine, 2006) reported on the factors that predicted treatment-seeking behaviour in a group of university students and staff with migraines. Two factors, social support and locus of control, were considered. Altogether 100 subjects who met the migraine criteria of the International Headache Society were included. Instruments to reflect the unique social support needs of headache sufferers included the Actually Received Support sub-scale of the Berlin Social Support Scales. The multi-dimensional Health Locus of Control Scale was used as the basis for the Headache Specific Locus of Control Scale.

The results were unequivocal in showing that, in their consulting behaviour, the help-seekers differed significantly from non-consulters on the Social Support Active Involvement sub-scale as well as the Healthcare Professional Locus of Control sub-scale. Attitudes concerning the role of healthcare professionals and a supportive social network were more powerful predictors of treatment-seeking behaviour than demographic characteristics, beliefs about medication, and headache severity and frequency.

The aspects-of-social-support scale included significant others (parent, spouse, children, friend, etc.) who were actively involved with the headache sufferer. Another element was the reaction of the significant other to the patient. Combined, these two components presented a comprehensive picture of the social support available to and used by the headache sufferers. The authors noted that an active involvement dimension of social support was found to significantly impact consulting behaviour. The presence of an active intimate did promote health-seeking behaviour. Further research with a larger population of migraine sufferers was recommended.

Summary

The four studies discussed above provided a complex picture of the use and benefits of social support by chronic headache sufferers in very different situations. The first study (Martin and Theunissen, 1993) using a relatively small sample of sufferers of migraine and chronic tension-type headaches found that headache sufferers differed significantly in their use of social support compared to the normal controls, and the data supported the proposition that lower social support was associated with higher stress levels. The second study (Vos & Passchier, 2003) was conducted with a large sample of 448 migraine sufferers, and demonstrated the use of a wide range of social support systems that seemed to suggest that problem-specific support was sought by the patients. The third study (Peters, Abu-Sadd, Robbins, Vydelingum, et al., 2005) examined the strategies used by migraine and daily headache sufferers (n=438) and found a rather low use of social support, although the authors noted that social support was part of a coping repertoire for a significant proportion (30%) of the patients. The final study (Skomo, Desselle, & Berdine, 2006) examined the treatment-seeking behaviour of a group of migraine sufferers (n=100), and reported that the active involvement of those who provide social support to the patients promoted treatment-seeking behaviour. These four studies varied in scope and objectives. Collectively, they did confirm the beneficial aspects of social support in very different circumstances.

The Downside of Social Support

The above phrase was used by Turk and colleagues to bring to the fore the notion that all social support may not always be beneficial (Turk, Kerns, & Rosenberg, 1992). On the contrary, certain types of social support can hinder the progress of patients. This idea is rooted in operant conditioning and was originally proposed by Fordyce (1976), who made the astute observation that a certain kind of pain-reinforcement behaviour by a spouse, albeit with good intentions, had unintended consequences. Turk and colleagues provided a succinct summary of this phenomenon: 'A solicitous spouse may unwittingly contribute to the patient's pain experience through the selective reinforcement of pain behaviors by provision of attention and sympathy for expression of pain and by passive sanctioning the avoidance of unwanted responsibilities or undesirable activities' (p. 262). A plethora of studies appeared in the scientific literature in support of the down side of social support or the operant model (Block, Kremer, & Gaylor, 1980; Flor, Turk, & Rudy, 1987; Gil, Keefe, Crisson, & Van Dalfsen, 1987; Kerns & Turk, 1984; Romano, Turner, Friedman, Bulcroft, et al., 1991). The fact that social support may not inevitably promote health and well-being was questioned in this sweeping reconsideration of the operant model. Turk and colleagues cautioned that more work was required to fully unravel the complexity of the power of spousal responses and the relationship of those responses to other factors that may profoundly influence pain, disability, and sadness. Romano and colleagues (1995) conducted a series of studies that provided further evidence in support of the proposition that solicitous spousal behaviour was generally associated with patients reporting more pain.

A decade later Newton-John (2002), in an exhaustive review of the literature, echoed some of the above sentiments. He analysed twenty-seven studies related to spouse–patient interaction, and found general support for the operant behavioural perspective. Nevertheless, he argued that this model alone excluded significant levels of complexity that were inherent in the spouse–patient relationship. One major conclusion reached was that the operant conditioning principles alone were not sufficient to account for the complexities inherent in couple relationships. Cognitive and affective variables need to be integrated into research programs. Chronic-pain couples' interactions were more complex than a purely behavioural model could accommodate. Newton-John further noted that there was emerging data to support the complex nature of marital interactions not entirely justified by the strictly behavioural perspective, as was noted by Roy (1985), and proposed further research to develop a broader understanding of the multifaceted nature of the spousal relationship.

In a more recent review, Leonard and associates (2006) confirmed that the empirical literature on couples and pain found validity for the operant perspective. Yet, there were several shortcomings. To date, only very limited evidence has emerged to support a relationship between marital satisfaction and perceived social support and pain variables. They also noted that marital satisfaction may have an indirect link with pain severity through the effect of these spouse responses. Further research was needed in the domain of pain acceptance, and of the variables, to better explain the relationship between spouse responses and other variables. This review, like the previous, also noted the interactional patterns that underlie the spousal relationship. Nevertheless, with the husbands of chronic pain sufferers, there was emerging data on loneliness, lower activity levels, greater subjective stress, and more fatigue than for husbands with pain-free wives. There were also reports of declining sexual and marital satisfaction. These and other factors may influence the spousal reinforcement of pain behaviours. Only further research will clarify their precise impact.

We end this section with recognition of the far-reaching consequences of the landmark book of Fordyce (1976). Without the foundation he laid down in *Behavioral methods in chronic pain and illness*, our current understanding of spousal pain-reinforcement behaviour, among other aspects, may not be as well understood. Patterson (2005) noted that the book 'has had a unique and indelible impact on the fields of pain, rehabilitation, and health psychology' (p. 314). He further observed that Fordyce's work created a new paradigm for treating chronic pain using operant approaches. Who can argue against that?

Summary

Fordyce (1976) proposed an elegant and yet simple idea that certain kind of (solicitous) behaviour in the spouse of a chronic pain sufferer is likely to have unintended consequences in that such behaviour may, in fact, reinforce a patient's pain behaviours, thus preventing progress. This proposition has been subjected to a remarkable amount of empirical research, which has, in large measure, confirmed it. The limitations of this proposition continue to further our understanding of the underlying complexities of spousal solicitous behaviour. The couple relationship is characterized by a multitude of social, psychological, ethnic, interpersonal, and other variables that must influence their interaction with each other. How these complex issues might influence spousal reinforcement behaviour remains a challenge for future researchers.

REFERENCES

[No author]. (2005). Management of chronic pain syndromes: Issues and interventions. *Pain Medicine, 6*, S1–S21.

Ahlberg-Hulten, G., Theorell, T., & Sigala, F. (1995). Social support, job-strain and musculo-skeletal pain among female healthcare personnel. *Scandinavian J. Work, Environment and Health, 21*, 435–439.

Bergman, S. (2005). Psychosocial aspects of chronic widespread pain and fibromyalgia. *Disability and Rehabilitation, 27*, 675–683.

Block, A., Kremer, E., & Gaylor, M. (1980). Behavioral treatment of chronic pain: The spouse as a discriminative cue for pain behavior. *Pain, 9*, 243–252.

Buenaver, L., Edwards, R., & Haythornthwaite, J. (2007). Pain-related catastrophizing and perceived social responses: Inter-relationships in the context of chronic pain. *Pain, 127*, 234–242.

Eriksen, W., Bruusgaard, D., & Knardahl, S. (2004). Work factors as predictors of intense or disabling low back pain: A prospective study of nurses' aides. *Occupational and Environmental Medicine, 61*, 398–404.

Feldman, S., & Downey, G. (1999). Pain, negative mood, and perceived support in chronic pain patients: A daily diary study of people with reflex sympathetic dystrophy syndrome. *J. Consulting & Clinical Psychology, 67*, 776–785.

Flor, H., Turk, D., & Rudy, T. (1987). The role of spouse reinforcement, perceived pain, and activity levels of chronic pain patients. *J. Psychosomatic Research, 31*, 251–259.

Fordyce, W. (1976). *Behavioral methods in chronic pain and illness*. St Louis: C.V. Mosby.

Gil, K., Keefe, F., Crisson, J., & Van Dalfsen, P. (1987) Social support and pain behavior. *Pain, 29*, 209–217.

Hoffman, P., Meier, B., & Council, J. (2002). A comparison of chronic pain between an urban and rural population. *J. Community Health Nursing, 19*, 213–224.

Jump, R., Robinson, M., Armstrong, A., Barnes, E., et al. (2005). Fatigue in systemic lupus erythematosus: Contribution of disease activity, pain, depression, and perceived social support. *J. Rheumatology, 32*, 1699–1705.

Kerns, R., & Turk, D. (1984). Depression and chronic pain: The mediating role of spouse. *J. Marriage and Family, 46*, 845–852.

Koleck, M., Mazaux, J., Rascle, N., & Bruchon-Schweitzer, M. (2006). Psychosocial factors and coping strategies as predictors of chronic evolution and quality of life in patients with low-back pain. *European J. Pain, 10*, 1–11.

Leonard, M., Cano, A., & Johanson, A. (2006). Chronic pain in a couples context: A review and integration of theoretical models and empirical evidence. *The J. Pain, 7*, 377–390.

Logerstrom, M., Wenemark, M., Hogberg, M., et al. (1995). Occupational and individual factors related to musculoskeletal symptoms in five body regions among Swedish nursing personnel. *Intl. Arch. Occup. Environ. Health, 68*, 27–35.

Lopez-Martinez, A., Esteve-Zarazaga, R., & Ramirez-Maestre, C. (2008). Perceived social support and coping responses are independent variables explaining pain adjustment among chronic pain patients. *The J. Pain, 9*, 373–379.

Martin, P., & Theunissen, C. (1993). The role of life-event stress and social support in chronic headache. *Headache, 33*, 301–306.

Newton-John, T. (2002). Solicitousness and chronic pain: A critical review. *Pain Reviews, 9*, 7–27.

Patel, S. (2007). Psychosocial predictors of pain chronicity in Navy servicemen. *Dissertation Abstracts International*, section B, *67* (7-B), pp. 4113.

Patterson, D. (2005). Behavioral methods for chronic pain and illness: A reconsideration and appreciation. *Rehabilitation Psychology, 50*, 312–315.

Peters, M., Abu-Sadd, H., Robbins, I., Vydelingum, V., Dowson, A., & Murphy, M. (2005). Patients' management of migraine and chronic daily headache: A study of the members of the Migraine Action Association (United Kingdom). *Headache, 45*, 571–581.

Reis, S., Hermoni, D., Borkan, J., Biderman, A., et al. (1999). A new look at low back complaints in primary care: A RAMBAM Israeli Family Practice Network Study. *J. Family Practice, 48*, 299–303.

Romano, J., Turner, J., Friedman, L., Bulcroft, R., et al. (1991). Observational assessment of chronic pain patient–spouse behavioral interaction. *Behavior Therapy, 22*, 549–567.

Roy, R. (1985). The interactional perspective behavior in marriage. *Int. J. Fam. Ther., 7*, 271–283.

Roy, R. (2001). *Social relations and chronic pain.* New York: Kluwer/Plenum.

Roy, R. (2007). Social dislocation and the chronic pain patient. In Michael Bond (Ed.), *Encyclopedia of Pain.* Heidelberg: Springer Verlag.

Ruehlman, L., Karoly, P., & Newton, C. (2008). Comparing the experiential and psychosocial dimensions of chronic pain in African Americans and Caucasians: Findings from a national community sample. *American Academy of Pain Medicine, 6*, 49–60.

Skomo, M., Desselle, S., & Berdine, H. (2006). Factors influencing migraineur-consulting behavior in a university population. *Headache, 46*, 742–749.

Tunks, E., Crook, J., & Weir, R. (2008). Epidemiology of chronic pain with psychosocial co-morbidity: Prevalence, risk, course, and prognosis. *Canadian J. Psychiatry, 53*, 224–234.

Tunks, E., Weir, R., & Crook, J. (2008). Epidemiologic perspective on chronic pain treatment. *Canadian J. Psychiatry, 53*, 235–242.

Turk, D., Kerns, R., & Rosenberg, R. (1992). Effects of marital interaction on chronic pain and disability: Examining the down side of social support. *Rehabilitation Psychology, 1*, 259–274.

Turner, J., Clancy, S., & Vitaliano, P. (1987). Relationship of stress, appraisal and coping, to chronic low back pain. *Behavior Research and Therapy, 25*, 281–288.

Vos, J., & Passchier, J. (2003). Reduced impact of migraine in everyday life: An observational study in the Dutch Society of Headache Patients. *Headache, 43,* 645–650.

Waxman, S., Tripp, D., & Flamenbaum, R. (2008). The mediating role of depression and negative partner response in chronic low-back pain and relationship satisfaction. *The J. Pain, 9,* 434–442.

Woods, V. (2005). Work-related musculoskeletal health and social support. *Occupational Medicine, 55,* 177–189.

5 Depression in Perspective

Introduction

Major depression (MD) is one of the most common psychiatric disorders. It is a complex and multidimensional disorder that is influenced, among other factors, by age, gender, education, income, and marital status. Epidemiologic data around the globe shows that MD is almost twice as common in women than men. A major Canadian epidemiologic study (Patten, Wang, Williams, Currie, et al., 2006) revealed that the lifetime prevalence of a major depressive episode was 12.2%; past-year episodes were 4.8% of the sample. The target population for this study was persons aged fifteen years and over living in private dwellings. The diagnostic criteria for major depression followed the DSM-IV criteria, with the exception of a duration requirement for a manic episode. The prevalence of major depression was unrelated to level of education, but was related to one's having a chronic medical condition, to unemployment, and to income. One critical finding, relevant to the topic at hand, was that the prevalence of major depressive disorder was greater in the unmarried group, and was two-thirds times higher for divorced and separated subjects. The risk of major depression increased with age. Women were more susceptible than men.

Ohayon (2006) investigated major depressive disorder in a sample of 6694 individuals aged between 18 and 96 years. This population was a representative sample of the general population of the states of California and New York. The one-month prevalence of major depressive disorder was 5.2% of the sample, with higher rates for female, middle aged, and non-Hispanic individuals. Factors such as age, being separated or divorced, and lower education had greater influence on prevalence rates than gender alone. These two reports not only confirm the relative commonness of major depression in the general population, but firmly demonstrate the complex interplay of psychosocial factors in the genesis of this disease.

The following paper (Desai & Jann, 2000) provides a major review of the literature of major depression in women. It is a very broad-based review of depression in women. We report the data they reported on the prevalence of major depression. First, worldwide, major depression is twice as common in women than in men. Second, major epidemiologic studies have consistently reported higher lifetime and one-year prevalence rates of major depression in women. The lifetime prevalence of depression in community samples varied from 10–25% in women, with an average prevalence of approximately 20%. By comparison, the lifetime prevalence in men was 5–12%, with an average of 10%. The male to female lifetime relative risk of a major depressive episode ranged from 1.7 to 2.4%.

We conclude this section with a recent Canadian study. Patten and Schopflocher (2009) conducted a community-based study to determine the epidemiology of major depression. Their sample of 3304 community residents was drawn from random digit dialling. Each subject had a baseline assessment using the 9-item Brief Patient Health Questionnaire (PGQ-9) followed by six subsequent interviews, six weeks apart.

The rate of prevalence was 2.5–3.5% during each interview. The incidence of new episodes was high, but many of the episodes were of brief duration. A high rate of recovery was observed at baseline, but declined over time. An anti-depressant was used by 11.1% at the baseline interview and remained stable over time. The PHQ-9 results indicated that many subjects had brief and perhaps time-limited episodes. PHQ-9, however, has not been an instrument of choice in epidemiological research on major depression. One major conclusion reached by this study was that 'the longstanding episodes (of major depression) typically encountered in clinical practice appear to represent a minority of occurrences of the major depressive syndromes in the community' (p. 31). PHQ-9, however, did not differentiate persistent or chronic depression from transient episodes. This finding, at least in part, explained why a proportion of subjects failed to seek treatment for episodes of major depression that were mostly reactive and of brief duration.

Summary

Major depression is a relatively common psychiatric condition that is more pervasive in women than men. The risk of major depression increases with age. Psychosocial factors, such as marital status, income, level of education, childhood abuse, gender, and age play a significant role in the etiology of this condition. Although there are some differences in the estimates of the rate of prevalence and incidence of major depression in the epidemiologic literature, there is broad agreement on the relative common occurrence of this condition in the general population. Our last study, despite its limitations due to sample selection and other methodological issues, demands more replication using the PHQ-9. One significant finding of this study is that while major depression is a relatively common disease, much of it is time-limited and does not require active medical intervention.

Depression and Marital Disruption

Marriage has been demonstrated to promote health (see the following section). In chapter 1 we found the power of an intimate relationship to prevent morbidity or hasten the process of recovery from illness. Therefore, we think it is important to consider that a marital relationship can cause harm resulting in depression. The relationship between depression and marital conflict is a complicated one. Marital disruption may lead to depression (Uebelacker & Wishman, 2005; Wishman & Uebelacker, 2009) and the reverse of that is equally true (Papp, Gocke Morey, & Cummings, 2007). This relationship is bidirectional (Davila, Karney, Hall, & Bradbury 2003). This phenomenon is well illustrated by two somewhat dated, but well-executed studies (O'Leary, Christian, & Mendell, 1994; Weissman, 1987). O'Leary and associates reported that in the face of marital conflict, the risk of depression increased tenfold. Weissman, in a major epidemiological study, found that risk for a major depression increased twenty-five-fold in unsatisfactory compared to satisfactory marriages.

The body of literature on this topic is rich and extensive. It is also a fact, as we discuss in the following section, that many psychological benefits accrue from marriage. We summarize next the key conclusions from three recent, exhaustive literature reviews on the relationship between marital distress and depression (Mead, 2002; Rehman, Gollan, & Mortimer, 2008; Wishman, 2001).

Mead, in his comprehensive review of marital distress and depression and marital therapy cited several authors to show that marital stress in the newly married was related to lack of social support for wives from their husbands, and that this was a product of the generation of stress, revealing a cyclical relationship between depressed mood in wives and support from husbands. Further, there was some evidence to suggest that marital relationship of poor quality predicted higher levels of depression in wives than in husbands. Mead also noted the bidirectional nature of the relationship between marital distress and depression. Data has shown that individuals who experienced depression in marriage probably had their first encounter with this condition at a much younger age. He drew attention to the high rate of divorce in persons with a history of depression. One estimate was that individuals with a history of major depression had a 70% greater probability for separation and divorce.

We have reported only a small part of this review that is directly relevant to the topic at hand. Nevertheless, it is worth noting that its scope was substantial, covering the following areas: mediators and moderators, that is, factors that mediate and moderate both depression and marital conflict; gender as a possible moderating factor; marital distress as a cause for depression; the impact of depression on a spouse; the role of social support; and the pharmacological treatment of depression. It also provided an exhaustive review of the couple therapy literature.

The next paper (Wishman, 2001) reported on a meta-analysis of the empirical literature on the association between depressive symptoms and marital dissatisfaction. Wishman conducted a meta-analysis across 26 studies involving more than 3700 women and 2700 men. Marital dissatisfaction accounted for approximately 18% of the variance in depressive symptoms in wives and 14% in husbands. The effect sizes ranged from medium to large. The association was significantly greater for women.

Wishman also examined the research literature on the long-term association between depression and marital dissatisfaction. His analysis yielded mixed findings. Generally, increases in depressive symptoms were accompanied by decreases in marital quality. The studies reviewed found that both depressive symptoms and dissatisfaction with marriage resulted in long-term change. Future research needed to focus on the trajectory of change in 'risk factors' for marital dissatisfaction, the trajectory of change in marital dissatisfaction, and the link between the two trajectories. Wishman's overall conclusion was that the existing literature found strong support for an association between marital dissatisfaction and depressive symptoms, and that women were at greater risk than men. Marital dissatisfaction may very well pre-date the onset of depression, and this effect may also be greater for women than men.

The focus of our final paper (Rehman, Gollan, & Mortimer, 2008) is the empirical research on the marital communication behaviours of depressed individuals. The authors write: 'Interpersonal perspectives of depression are important as they provide a framework to understand the impact of depression on the lives of people who live with the depressed individual. Studies have shown that living with a depressed spouse has been associated with negative outcomes for the non-depressed spouse' (p. 181).

In discussing the bidirectional nature of the temporal relationship between depression and marital conflict, Rehman and associates (2008) noted that a shift has occurred in the focus of research that explores the reciprocal influences of depression and marital distress. New statistical techniques for analysing multi-wave data make it possible to conduct a within-subject analysis of the complex and dynamic nature of the relationship between depression and marital conflict. The bidirectional relationship may have components that help determine the outcome. In conclusion, Rehman and colleagues make a case for a change in the direction of research, which needs to have strong theoretical underpinnings, and help identify the methodological and conceptual limitations of the existing research literature.

Summary

That there is an association between marital dissatisfaction and depression has received strong empirical support. There is also evidence for depression causing marital conflict. Women are at greater risk for depression when confronted with an unhappy marriage. The long-term relationship between the two factors and the nature of the temporal relationship remain somewhat unclear. There is also recognition that the marital relationship is complex, and the research methods employed to date have not adequately captured this complexity.

Benefits of Marriage

Our brief excursion into the epidemiology of pain revealed a positive relationship between marriage and the absence of depression and that separated and divorced individuals were more at risk for this condition. We now provide a brief overview of that topic. Mead (2002) observed that marriage was known to insulate both women and men from depression. Waite and Gallagher (2000), citing another study, found that married people, with and without children, were healthier than their single counterparts. Marriage has also been associated with better health and longevity (Coyne & Benazon, 2001). Yet, family is also recognized as a major source of many interpersonal, including marital, conflicts (Roy, 2006). In this section, we examine the power of the marital/partner relationship to prevent or mitigate depression and the cost of the absence of such a relationship.

Much empirical evidence has also emerged documenting the positive relationship between a transition to marriage and general psychological well-being (Simon & Marcussen, 1999; Simon, 2002; Williams, 2006). Stack and Eshleman (1998) conducted a remarkable study to investigate marital status and happiness in seventeen industrialized countries. The study's purpose was simple: to explore whether the phenomenon of an association between marital status and happiness was cross-cultural. The authors noted that three intermediating processes accounted for the impact of marital status on personal well-being. Marriage is thought to affect well-being by increasing financial resources, fostering better physical health, and providing better emotional support.

Data for this study was collected during 1981–3 from the World Values Study Group. Complete data sets were available on 18,000 adults from seventeen countries. Happiness was measured quite simply by asking if the respondents were: not at all happy; not very happy; quite happy; or very happy. The authors warned about the limitations of single-item measures. The results showed that married persons reported significantly more happiness than did single persons. The variable that accounted for most happiness was satisfaction with household finance, followed by health status. Emotional support was not a significant factor.

In sixteen out of seventeen countries, marital status was significantly related to happiness. The strength of the relationship between being married and happiness was consistent across the nations. Furthermore, there was no gender difference concerning marital status and happiness. The authors cautioned that one major limitation of the study was that it was confined to mostly Western, industrially developed nations. These findings may or may not be relevant to countries that fall outside the somewhat narrow scope of this study.

French and Williams (2007) conducted a study to demonstrate the benefits of marriage for a group of subjects with and without depression. Their sample was derived from the National Survey of Families and Households. Their first sample was restricted to those unmarried at Time 1 and married at Time 2. Valid instruments were used to collect data on psychological well-being, marital transition, and marital quality. Respondents over the age of fifty-five were excluded, as were respondents with missing psychological data. The final sample consisted of 3066 cases.

The results showed that those who were depressed before marrying experienced greater benefits than those who were not depressed. The authors provided many plausible explanations for this finding, among them the possibility that marriage furnished a level of companionship that a depressed person needed, unlike for a non-depressed individual. Noteworthy was the fact that the previously depressed had slightly but significantly worse marital happiness than the non-depressed. Overall, male and female subjects reported rather similar patterns in the relationships among prior depression, the transition to marriage, and psychological well-being. The authors cautioned that the mechanisms through which premarital levels of depression and single-person status affect the psychological benefits of marriage are not well comprehended.

Cairney, Boyle, Offord, and Racine (2003) investigated the effects of stress and social support on the relationship between single-parent status and depression. The sample of single and married mothers was drawn from the general population. The results showed that compared to married mothers, single mothers were more likely to have suffered an episode of depression, to have experienced a higher level of chronic stress, to have had more recent life-events, and to have experienced a greater number of childhood adversities. The analysis showed that for depression in the single mothers, stress and (lack of) social support accounted for 40% of the relationship between single-parent status and depression. A major conclusion to be drawn from the study was that marriage appeared to have had a measurable buffering function against depression.

Marital breakdown, while common in today's society, is still a major cause of psychological distress. Bruce and Kim (1992) investigated depression in a population of men and women who had separated or divorced and compared them with both 'happily married' and 'not getting along with their spouse' subjects. The key finding was that the prevalence rates of major depression were higher in men and women experiencing marital disruption compared to the happily married. Men were at a higher risk for a first onset of major depression than women. The authors noted that these findings were consistent with previous findings reporting that the advantages of marriage were greater for men than for women. Women, by contrast, tend to experience depression earlier in the course of marriage difficulties than men. One major omission of this study was that the design did not permit the timing of the marital disruption with the onset of the major depressive episode. This omission is of considerable import, as there is generally a temporal relationship between occurrence of an event and the onset of symptoms.

There also exists a body of research studies showing the benefits, including recovery from depression, that accrue from separation and divorce (Aseltine & Kessler, 1993; Cohen, Klein, & O'Leary, 2007; Green, 1983; Wheaton, 1990). These four studies reported a reduction in depressive symptoms (in subjects already suffering from clinical depression and/or difficulties in marriage) following divorce. We discuss briefly the findings of Cohen and colleagues, who examined the impact of separation/divorce on the course of depression in a group of subjects who experienced their first encounter with major depression at age twenty-two. The sample included a combination of both currently depressed (n=22) and recovered (n=22) individuals at the point of marriage dissolution. Subjects who were depressed at the time of marital dissolution had a five-fold increase in the probability of recovery from their depressive illness relative to subjects who did not. Subjects who were not depressed at the time of marital breakdown failed to show any significant risk for a relapse. The authors concluded that their study provided 'empirical support for the position that the effects of divorce appear to be diminished and/or absent for individuals who experience the end of their marriage as an escape rather than a loss' (Cohen, Klein, & O'Leary, 2007, p. 857).

The idea that marriage almost inevitably leads to happiness and better health and prosperity has come under some scrutiny (Hui, 2008; Williams, 2006). Hui conducted a comprehensive analysis of the literature on marital status and health differentials from the 1970s to the 2000s. The results failed to confirm the long-standing support for the belief in the positive relationship between marriage and health. In fact, the self-rated health of the never-married began to resemble that of the married. In contrast, over the same time span, the self-rated health of the widowed, divorced, and separated worsened compared to that of the married. The author also questioned the evidence that family income explained the health trends by marital status. Important gender and race variations in health trends by marital status and some long-held views about gender, marital status, and health were also challenged.

Williams (2006) explored the extent to which intimate relationships produced positive outcome for African American professional women. The question Williams sought to answer was whether these women were psychologically healthier than African American professional single women. A variety of standardized instruments were used to assess the health and psychological well-being of the subjects.

The results showed that significant differences did exist in the domain of loneliness between the partnered women and single women. A correlation analysis showed that coping resources were associated with self-esteem for African American single women, and the number of years in a long-term relationship was associated with depression. The importance of marriage was related to self-esteem, and coping resources were correlated with loneliness for African American partnered women. Overall, both groups exhibited psychological well-being regardless of their marital status. The author concluded that for this sample of women, being highly educated, being in established careers, and having financial independence may explain their overall psychological well-being. In short, the factors associated with high social economic status levelled off the benefits of marriage or partnership.

Summary

The first three studies discussed here addressed three very different aspects of marriage. Married persons seemed to be less prone to suffer from major depression, and one conclusion from that body of literature was that marriage served a preventive function in that married individuals were less susceptible to depression.

Single parenthood, which in Canada is associated with a high rate of poverty, presents many and varied challenges, one of which is a risk for depression. Marital disruption and difficulties is another source of distress, and the literature suggests that this may be another source of depression. In this category of studies, women rather than men also are more vulnerable for major depression. However, it is clear from another body of research illustrated in the study by Cohen and associates (2007) that the conditions under which marital breakdown happens is a predictor of the susceptibility to depression.

Divorce or separation from stressful marriages can seemingly help individuals recover from depression. Our last two studies, however, pose serious questions about the inevitability of the benefits of marriage. Many factors may indeed influence the health outcome in single persons. High socio-economic status, changing family patterns such as people choosing to stay single (31% of the households in Canada are one-person households) (Roy 2006), and other social and economic factors may have significant modifying effects on the health outcome of single people. In the section that follows we examine the broad literature on the relationship between social support and major depression. Acknowledging that the research literature on social support and depression is truly vast, we present what must be considered a very small fraction of it. Following a general discussion of this topic, we examine the power of social support in middle-aged and older subjects.

Effectiveness of Social Support and Clinical Depression

Brown and Harris (1978) in their seminal book provided a comprehensive understanding of the role of social support in the genesis of depression in women. They proposed that low levels of support could create a sense of failure and unhappiness leading to formation of low self-esteem, which in turn left the individual vulnerable to the negative consequences of stressful life-events. These events often involved some kind of loss. In general terms, individuals with low self-esteem experiencing severe losses were also more likely to develop clinical depression. The theory underlying the above proposition is rooted in the vulnerability model of social support.

Vilhjalmsson (1993) in her elegant and comprehensive re-analysis of social-support and clinical-depression literature made a number of important points. First, she pointed out the three mechanisms for interaction between social support and clinical depression: (1) support exclusively modified stress, which prevented the harmful consequences of stress; (2) support still acted totally as a stress modifier, but failed to buffer stress; and (3) stress and support probably had only marginal effect on mental health.

In her re-analysis of twelve community-based studies, she reached a major conclusion that their analyses of the effects of stress and social support on clinical depression were filled with inconsistent results. Individual studies had inconsistent statistical power. While eight out of twelve studies explained the data with only main effects, it did not necessarily mean that the idea of stress modification was rejected. The critical question this reviewer attempted to answer was whether social support was a stress modifier (vulnerability model) or an independent causal agent (strain model) in clinical depression. On the basis of her re-analysis, Vilhjalmsson concluded that the strain model provided a better explanation for the relationship between social support and clinical depression. She also noted that the results of her finding were not generalizable due to the fact that most studies on clinical depression were restricted to women's support from their husbands, cohabitants, or boy friends. Vilhjalmsson made an important contribution (1) by raising fundamental questions about the underlying theory that might explain the power of social support in moderating or preventing clinical depression and (2) by re-analysing existing studies to find significant methodological issues, which led to reformulating some of the original findings.

Olstad, Sexton, and Sogaard (2001), in a community-based study in Finnmark, Norway, involving 2250 subjects with a maximum of 5409 observations, tested the buffer hypothesis of social support or the social network and mental health. The ages of the subjects ranged from 40 to 60 years; a random sample of those aged between 20 and 39 years were invited to participate in the three health surveys. The General Health Questionnaire was used to assess mental health (depression). Subjects were asked if they were depressed over the period of the previous two weeks. Social support was divided into instrumental support, which was measured by the extent to which the subjects borrowed things from their neighbours, received help with transport, in repairing things, or in looking after house while subject was away, and the answers were ranged from 'Never' to 'Often.' Emotional support consisted of talking to family members or someone outside the family about joys, sorrows, or health issues during the previous two weeks, and the responses consisted of Yes/No.

The results were complex. Overall, when all possible stressors and entirety of the social network or social support were analysed, there was clear evidence that social support did buffer the negative effects on mental health from all stressors. Although the effect was weak, it was still significant. The social network had a significant buffering effect in work situations. The buffering effect of social support and the social network was most evident among persons receiving a disability pension.

The authors concluded that having a good total social network/ support weakly buffered the deteriorating effect of total stress on depression. This was an important study for several reasons. It was a prospective study with a large community-based population. A standardized instrument was used to measure depression, and a complex system to assess social network/support. The study was very specific about the situations where social network/support was effective. This study found weak and specific support for the buffering hypothesis in relation to network and social support and depression.

Matud, Carballeira, et al. (2002), in a large community-based study (n=2169) on the relationship between social support and health for both men, and women, reported that low social support was strongly correlated with somatic symptoms, anxiety and insomnia, social dysfunction and severe depression. Women were more vulnerable, than men except in the domain of somatic symptoms and social dysfunction. Socio-demographic variables produced only weak relationships , but were statistically significant only for women. Education and the level of social support were positively related. Gender differences also emerged in relation to married subjects. Professional subjects had more social support than manual workers. Homemakers had lower social support than non-manual female workers and professionals. This paper confirmed a number of known facts and illuminated others further. One example of that in relation to gender was the finding that women were more vulnerable than men to somatic symptoms and social dysfunction. The role of occupation and education as important determinants for the availability of social support received further confirmation.

Our next three studies involve social support and major depression, comparing middle-aged with older adults (George, Blazer, Hughes, & Fowler, 1989), gender differences in opposite twin sex pairs (Kendler, Myers, & Prescott, 2005), and the buffering effect of social support in relation to the elderly (Hays, Steffens, Flint, Bosworth, & George, 2001). George and colleagues compared 150 middle-aged (30–50 years) and older (than 60) subjects with a diagnosis of major depression for their subjective assessment of social support while in-patients at the Duke University Center. Patients were assessed for their response to the treatment of depression, life-events, and social support. The size of the social network and subjective social support were significant predictors of depressive symptoms at follow-up. Subjective social support was most strongly related to major depression in the middle-age group and more for men than women.

The results of this study found strong support for the hypothesis that social support has a determining effect on the outcome of depressive illness. The strongest and the most complex relationship emerged between subjective social support and depression. Authors concluded that the differences in the effects of marital status, size of social network, and subjective social support point up the importance of differentiating between involvement in and the quality of interpersonal relationships. This was a complex study examining the power of perceived social support to predict the outcome of depressive illness. The main-effect model of social support received confirmation in relation to subjective social support and outcome.

Kendler and colleagues (2005), in an unique study, conducted an investigation to examine the relationship between baseline levels of social support and the risk for future episodes of major depression. The subjects for this study consisted of opposite-sex twin pairs drawn from the Virginia Adult Twin Study of Psychiatric and Substance Abuse Disorders.

In waves of interviews one year apart, 1057 pairs of opposite-sex dizygotic twins were assessed for social support and major depression. The results were unequivocal in showing that women scored higher levels of social support than their twin brothers. Global social support at wave 1 predicted major depression at wave 2 significantly more strongly in women than in men in these pairs. Women were more sensitive than men to depression-inducing effects of low levels of social support, especially from the co-twin, other relatives, parents, and spouses. The levels of social support, however, failed to explain the sex differences in risk for major depression. These effects do explain, in part, sex differences in pathways of risk. The authors concluded that interpersonal relationships were more central to and more valued by women than men. In difficult circumstances, women were more likely to seek emotional social support than men. This study provided powerful evidence of a strong 'direct effect of social support on risk for major depression' (p. 254).

Our final study in this section (Hays et al., 2001) tested the buffering model of social support and its power to protect against functional decline in elderly patients with unipolar depression. The patients for this study were drawn from the Mental Health Clinical Research

Center for the Study of Depression in Later Life at Duke University. The patients included in this study were limited to those with unipolar major depression. Those with other psychiatric disorders, alcohol or drug dependency, neurological problems, or other medical conditions were excluded.

Altogether 113 subjects (mean age 69.5 years) were followed up for 12 months while undergoing the required treatment. They were tested on the performance of instrumental activities of daily living, a measure of depression, and four domains (size of social network, amount of social interaction, availability of instrumental aid, and subjective social support) of informal social support. The results showed that the subjects improved on their instrumental activities and remained stable on the basic activities of daily living. Large social networks, more frequent social interactions, and the perceived adequacy of social support played a buffering role, albeit modest, against decline in performance in the basic activities of daily living among the most severely depressed elderly patients.

This study tested the three following hypothesis: (1) that depressive symptoms would predict functional declines 1 year, a hypothesis that received strong support; (2) that social support would mitigate the effect of depression severity of functional declines at 1 year, which was only modestly supported; and (3) that the buffering effects of social support against functional decline would be strongest among the most severely depressed patients, which received only partial support. Overall, social support had only a modest effect on maintaining or restoring the functional abilities of a group of elderly patients with unipolar depression

Summary

Our sojourn into the research literature on social support and depression reveals one central fact. As the methodology has improved over the years, the findings have become more and more complex. Vilhjalmsson (1993) concluded that research had failed to convincingly demonstrate that social support had a moderating effect on depression. In fact, two more recent studies (Skarsater, Argen, and Dencker, 2001; Wade & Kendler, 2000) provided more insight into this complex relationship. Wade and Kendler found little evidence for the power of social support to mitigate major depression. Skarsater and associates concluded that patients with major depression, compared to a control group of healthy volunteers, were exposed to more stressful events, and they had more arguments with their intimates such as partners and family members. Sources of social support turned into sources for distress. In the studies discussed above only one (George, Blazer, Hughes, and Fowler 1989) found strong support for the buffering model. The rests of the studies reported more complex findings, at best finding a weak case for the buffering power of social support either to mitigate depression or to predict better outcome.

Conclusion

The literature on the various aspects of major depression and social support that we have addressed above is truly voluminous. We have presented a highly selected and small part of that body of literature. Major depression is a relatively common disorder which affects women more than men. Marriage has its benefits, but it also has a darker side. Conflict in marriages impacts quite negatively on mental health, again mostly on wives. Husbands, however, are not immune to the adverse effects of bad marriages.

There is greater recognition that the marital relationship is complex, and this complexity has not been captured by research. There is call for methodologically improved research. Social support does influence the outcome of depression in a positive way, but the research findings are more complicated. The buffering model of social support has proved to have limited value. Social support has been shown to have only a modest buffering effect on major depression.

REFERENCES

Aseltine, R., & Kessler, R. (1993). Marital disruption and depression in a community sample. *J. Health Social Behav., 34*, 237–251.

Brown, G., & Harris, T. (1978). *Social origins of depression: A study of psychiatric disorder in women.* New York: The Free Press.

Bruce, M., & Kim, K. (1992). Differences in the effects of divorce on major depression in men and women. *Am. J. Psychiatry, 149,* 914–917.

Cairney, J., Boyle, M., Offord, D., & Racine, Y. (2003). Stress, social support and depression in single and married mothers. *Social Psychiatry and Psychiatric Epidemiology, 38*: 442–449.

Cohen, S., Klein, D., & O'Leary, D. (2007). The role of separation/divorce in relapse into and recovery from major depression. *J. Social & Personal Relationship, 24*, 855–873.

Coyne, J., & Benazon, N. (2001). Not agent blue: Effects of marital functioning on depression and implications for treatment. In S. Beach (Ed.), *Marital and family processes in depression: Scientific processes for clinical practice*. Washington, DC: American Psychological Association.

Davila, J., Karney, B., Hall, T., & Bradbury, T. (2003). Depressive symptoms and marital satisfaction: Within-subjects associations and the moderating effects of gender and neuroticism. *J. Family Psychology, 17*: 457–470.

Desai, H., & Jann, M. (2000). Major depression in women: A review of the literature. *J. American Pharmacists Association, 40*, 525–537.

French, A., & Williams, K. (2007). Depression and the psychological benefits of entering marriage. *J. Health & Social Behavior, 48*, 149–163

George, L., Blazer, D., Hughes, D., & Fowler, N. (1989). Social support and outcome of major depression. *Br. J. Psychiatry, 154*, 478–485.

Green, R. (1983). The influence of divorce prediction variables on divorce adjustment: An expansion and test of Lewis and Spanier's theory of marital quality and marital stability. *J. Divorce, 7*, 67–81.

Hays, J., Steffens, D., Flint, E., Bosworth, H.. & George, L. (2001). Does social support buffer functional decline in elderly patients with unipolar depression. *Am. J. Psychiat., 158*, 1850–1855.

Hui, L. (2008). The times they are a changin': Marital status and health differentials from the 1970s to 2000s. *Dissertation Abstracts International*, section A, *69* (6A).

Kendler, K., Myers, J., & Prescott, C. (2005). Sex differences in the relationship between social support and risk for major depression: A longitudinal study of opposite sex twin pairs. *Am. J. Psychiat., 162*, 250–256.

Matud, P., Carballeira, M., Lopez, M., Marrero, R., & Ibanez, I. (2002). Social support and health: A gender analysis. *Salud Mental* [Spanish], *25*: 32–37.

Mead, D. (2002). Marital distress, co-occurring depression, and marital therapy: A review. *J. Marital & Family Therapy, 28*, 299–314.

Ohayon, M. (2006). Epidemiology of depression and its treatment in the general population. *J. Psychiatric Research, 41*, 207–213.

O'Leary, K., Christian, J., & Mendell, N. (1994). A closer look at the link between marital discord and depressive symptomatology. *J. Social & Clinical Psychology, 13*, 33–41.

Olstad, R., Sexton, H., & Sogaard, A. (2001). The Finnmark Study: A prospective population study of the social support buffer hypothesis, specific stressor and mental health. *Soc. Psychiat Psychiatric Epidemiology, 36*, 582–589.

Papp, L., Goeke-Morey, M., & Cummings, E. (2007). Linkages between spouses' psychological distress and marital conflict in the home. *J. Family Psychology, 21*, 533–537.

Patten, S., & Schopflocher, D. (2009). Longitudinal epidemiology of major depression as assessed by the Brief Patient Health Questionnaire (PHQ-9). *Comprehensive psychiatry, 50*, 26–33.

Patten, S., Wang, J., Williams, J., Currie, S., et al. (2006). Descriptive epidemiology of major depression in Canada. *Canadian. J. Psychiatry, 51*, 84–90.

Rehman, U., Gollan, J., & Mortimer, A. (2008). The marital context of depression: Research, limitations, and new directions. *Clinical Psychology Review, 28*, 179–198.

Roy, R. (2006). *Chronic pain and family: A clinical perspective.* New York, Springer.

Simon, R. (2002). Revisiting the relationships between gender, marital status, and mental health. *American J. Sociology, 107*, 111–125.

Simon, R., & Marcussen, K. (1999). Marital transitions, marital beliefs, and mental health. *J. Health & Social Behavior, 40*, 111–125.

Skarsater, I., Argen, H., & Dencker, K. (2001). Subjective lack of social support and presence of dependent stressful life events characterize patients suffering from major depression compared to healthy volunteers. *J. Psychiat. Mental Health Nursing, 8*, 107–114.

Stack, S., & Eshleman, R. (1998). Marital status and happiness: A 17-nation study. *J. Marriage & Family, 60*, 527–536.

Uebelacker, L., & Wishman, M. (2005). Relationship beliefs, attributions, and partner behaviors among depressed married women. *Cognitive Therapy & Research, 29*: 143–154.

Vilhjalmsson, R. (1993). Life stress, social support and clinical depression: A re-analysis of literature. *Soc. Sc. Med., 37*: 331–342.

Wade, T., & Kendler, K. (2000). Absence of interactions between social support and stressful life events in the prediction of major depression and depressive symptomatology in women. *Psychological Medicine, 30*, 965–974.

Waite, L., & Gallagher, M. (2000). *The case for marriage: Why married people are healthier, happier, and better off financially.* New York: Doubleday.

Weissman, M. (1987). Advances in clinical epidemiology: Rates and risk of major depression. *Am. J. Public Health, 77*, 445–451.

Wheaton, B. (1990). Life transition, role histories, and mental health. *Am. Sociological Rev., 55*: 209–223.

Williams, N. (2006). The influence of intimate relationship on the psychological well-being of African-American professional women. *Dissertation Abstracts International*, section B, *66* (8-B).

Wishman, M. (2001). The association between depression and marital dissatisfaction. In S. Beach (Ed.), *Marital and family processes in depression: A scientific foundation for clinical practice*. Washington: American Psychological Association.

Wishman, M., & Uebelacker, L. (2009). Prospective associations between marital discord and depressive symptoms in middle-aged and older adults. *Psychology and Aging, 24*: 184–189.

6 Dementia and Social Support: Who Cares for the Caregivers?

In the United States an estimated 4.5 million persons have dementia, with an anticipated increase to 13.2 million by 2050 (Hebert, Scherr, Bienias, et al., 2003). The elderly population (over age 65) is expected to double from today's population of nearly 35 million to 70 million in 2030 (Plassman et al., 2007). With this rising population, a large number of them with dementia, programs for prevention and treatment of the chronic diseases of aging will assume increasing significance. A common occurrence of old age, dementia is associated with failing memory, loss of independence, and serious implications for the individuals' families, and the social and healthcare systems. Besides, behavioural and psychological problems are endemic to dementia.

A recent report by the Alzheimer's Society (2009) reported that Alzheimer's disease (AD) is the sixth leading cause of death in the United States. The estimate is that some 5.3 million Americans suffer from AD. Every 70 seconds someone in the United States is diagnosed with AD, and the estimates suggest that by 2050 this frequency will be increased to 33 seconds. Over the coming decade 10 million more Americans will fall prey to AD.

Plassman and colleagues (2007) reported the prevalence of dementia in a nationally representative sample of 856 individuals 71 years and older. The prevalence in this population was 13.9%. Prevalence of dementia increased with age, from 5% of those aged between 7 and 79, to 37.4% of those aged 90 years and over. They noted: 'As the US population grows, the number of individuals with dementia will also increase, making planning for the long-term care needs of these individuals increasingly important ... The first study of dementia in a nationally representative sample in the USA, extends beyond just estimating the prevalence of dementia to being able to address many of the key questions in preparing for the care of the demented and their families' (p. 130).

Lindsay, Sykes, McDowell, et al. (2004) in a review highlighted the contributions of the Canadian Study of Health and Aging, reporting the finding of the study, which began in 1991, with follow-ups in 1996 and 2001. The analysis involved 10,263 participants from 18 study centres. Of these, 9008 were in the community, and 1255 were in institutions. The study was conducted in three stages. In each phase participants were screened for cognitive impairment, and if necessary, their cognitive status was determined by a comprehensive medical examination. Risk factors were assessed on the initial contact.

The prevalence of dementia was found to be at 8% of those aged 65 and over, and incidence was about 2% each year. Prevalence rate rose 'dramatically' with age to 11.1% between the ages of 75 and 84, and 34.5% in those 85 years and older. Because of longevity in women their rate of dementia was more than double. Physical activity seemed to exert significant preventive power over all forms of dementia. Some of the risk factors associated with AD were increasing age, lower education, and the apoEe4 allele.

This study had several clinical implications, such as the development of neuropsychological tests for the cognitively normal population of persons 65 years and over, which made it possible to recognize normal cognitive aging. The protective effects of physical activity on the risk of cognitive impairment and dementia also had implications. However, further research was needed to corroborate this finding.

Our final study (Sawa, Zaccai, Matthews, Davidson, et al., 2009) reported the prevalence of behavioural and psychological symptoms associated with dementia (BPSD). The authors were associated with the Medical Research Council Cognitive Function and Aging Study (England and Wales), which offered a setting that managed to overcome some of the common problems associated with investigating the epidemiology of the behavioural and psychological problems of dementia.

In this study the authors described the epidemiology of BPSD in the elderly population of England and Wales. They estimated the prevalence of 12 symptoms in 587 study participants diagnosed with dementia at baseline, compared with similar symptoms in 2050 participants without dementia. The study population was followed up (with variations) at years 2, 6, 8, and 10. This study investigated the prevalence, co-occurrence, risk factors, and course of BPSD using a large representative sample of the population of England and Wales over 65 years. This was compared with the prevalence of the same symptoms in the population without dementia. The behavioural and psychological symptoms found in the BPSD were significantly less in the healthy sample with the exception of those affected by sleep disturbance. Major differences in the prevalence of the following symptoms between patients with dementia and without were as follows : apathy (50.3% vs 12.1%), irritability (28.8% vs 12.8%), feelings of persecution (25.4% vs 8.1%), depression (20.5% vs 8.6%), and misidentification (20.3% vs 3.0%). Significant differences were also found in hallucinations, wandering, elation, agitation, anxiety, and confabulation. Nevertheless, a significant proportion of the population without dementia also had disorders of mood, apathy, irritability, and feelings of persecution. The number of risk factors, such as the clinical and demographic, affected the presence of symptoms. Individual circumstances also had some influence. Most symptoms present at baseline were also likely to be present at the year-2 follow-up, although the strength of this association varied across symptoms.

Summary

Baby boomers entering their senior years at an ever-increasing pace will inevitably raise the proportion of the population who will be more susceptible to dementia. The epidemiology of dementia attests to that. This fact has enormous social, economic, and health policy consequences. In the rest of this chapter, we address one issue that confronts this group of our elderly citizens, which is the availability of support systems which may have beneficial results as they progress through this very overwhelming and often fatal condition(s). We shall discuss, first, the burden of caregiving; second, depression in caregivers; and third, the effectiveness of social support. We also note that due to the sheer volume of research literature related to our topic, we focus on the more recent literature, mostly of the last decade.

Caregiver Burden

The caregivers of patients with dementia are vulnerable to a multitude of stressors, in large part owing to the very nature of dementia. This is further complicated by the relationship quality and the age of the caregivers. Spousal support is perhaps the most common of all supports, and often because of the age of onset (usually advanced) of dementia, spouses themselves are older and not infrequently confronted with health problems. It is noteworthy that not just morbidity but also mortality has been associated with the caregivers (Vitaliano, Zhang, & Scanlan, 2003; Schulz & Beach, 1999). Mausbach, von Kanel, et al. (2007) conducted a study to determine the health effects of caregiving for the spouses of patients with Alzheimer's disease. An annual in-home assessment of plasma t-PA antigen were collected from 112 caregivers and 53 non-caregivers. Participants were married, were living with their spouses, were at least 55 years of age, and did not have any serious medical condition. The results were unequivocal. Caregivers showed significantly elevated increases in t-PA antigen over the five-year study period compared with the non-caregiving controls. The authors concluded that the accelerated rate of developing a prothrombotic environment including elevated t-PA antigen could be one mechanism which made the caregivers more vulnerable to greater morbidity and mortality and the development of cardiovascular disease. The caregivers of dementia patients tend to die prematurely due to strain, and a variety of mechanisms have been associated to explain this phenomena. The point is that the evidence of higher risk of morbidity and mortality for the caregivers of dementia patients is such that they deserve practical and emotional support to mitigate some of those risks. The poor health of caregivers also has profound implications for patients who depend on their intimates for support.

In a Spanish study, Serrano-Aguliar and colleagues (2006) noted that nearly 80% of individuals with AD are cared for at home by their family members. Their investigation revealed that the caregiver burden measured by the Zarit Burden Interview of 237 informal caregivers in their study was very high for 83.3% of their subjects. One central finding was that on the five dimensions (mobility; personal; daily activities; pain and discomfort; and anxiety/depression) of the Health Related Quality of Life (HQRL) measures, caregivers scored significantly higher on all five dimensions compared to the general population. The authors concluded: 'Taking care of an individual with Alzheimer's disease at home places high demands on caregivers with different and continuing problems as the disease progresses' (p. 139).

In a recent review of the research literature on the impact of the quality of the relationship with the care recipient on the well-being of caregivers Quinn, Clare, and Woods (2009) observed that the quality of the relationship prior to the onset of dementia does impact that relationship. These authors based their review on fifteen quantitative studies. This was an exhaustive review with multiple findings. We report some of their broad findings. First and foremost, there was ample evidence to support the proposition that caregiving can influence the quality of the relationship between the caregiver and care recipient. There was empirical support as well for the fact that the relationship quality could impact on the well-being of caregivers and on the care that they provided. However, there was very scanty evidence regarding the impact on relationship quality on the care recipient's well-being.

Some of the more specific findings were that caregivers with depression (a subject for the following section) had lower overall satisfaction with their marriage and their perceptions of marital cohesiveness. The quality of relationship was related to the levels of behavioural disturbance in the patient. Higher levels of marital intimacy was related to fewer behavioural disturbances. Gender and background factors also influenced the quality. Wives rated their prior relationship with care recipients less favourably than did their husbands. One important conclusion to emerge from this review was that caregivers who were married only once reported significantly higher levels of quality of life, less depression, better health, and more satisfaction with social relationships than caregivers married more than once. Another related finding was that higher quality of relationship was found when the care recipients were older, female, less educated, and had lower income.

The caregiver burden has been studied from multiple perspectives, which include comparing two types of dementia (Aalten, Tibben, et al., 2006), patient characteristics (Van Den Wijngaart, Vernoorij-Dassen, & Felling, 2007), caregiver characteristics (Sink, Covinsky, Barnes, Newcomer, and Yaffe, 2006; Vellone, Piras, Talucci, & Cohen, 2007), family (Mitrani, Lewis, Feaster, Czaja, et al., 2006), and cultural differences (Agulia, Onor, Trevisiol, Negro, et al., 2004; Nomura, Inoue, Shimodera, et al., 2005; Pang, Chow, Cummings, Leung, et al., 2002; Salgureo, Kohn, Salgureo, & Marotta, 1998).

We present a brief summary of the key findings on caregiver characteristics. One study investigated the relationship between caregiver characteristics and its relationship with the neuropsychiatric symptoms associated with dementia (Sink, Covinsky, Barnes, Newcomer, and Yaffe, 2006). This study was based on 5788 patients and their caregivers. Caregivers were asked about the presence of 12 neuropsychiatric symptoms in patients with dementia. The average age of the caregivers was 64 years; 72% were females. Spouses made up almost half (49%)

the caregivers. The patients were on average 79 years old. The key findings were that those caregivers who were less educated, younger, more depressed, more burdened, and reported more hours caring for the patient also reported more neuropsychiatric symptoms in their charges. The authors concluded that 'clinicians should consider the dynamics between patients and their caregivers when managing neuropsychiatric symptoms. Understanding how different caregiver characteristics influence neuropsychiatric symptoms may help tailor caregiver education and interventions' (Sink, Covinsky, et al., 2006, p. 796).

Allegri and associates (2006) investigated the predictive value of neuropsychiatric symptoms on the caregivers. The subjects consisted of 82 patients with probable Alzheimer's disease and their primary caregivers. They found that the presence of neuropsychiatric symptoms such as delusions, hallucinations, anxiety, euphoria, disinhibition, unusual motor behaviour, sleep disturbance, and changes in appetite were the best predictors for caregiver burden.

Vellone and associates (2007), in an investigation of 32 caregivers drawn from the gerontology department of a hospital in Rome, reported that caregivers identified the attributes that would provide a good quality of life: serenity, tranquillity, psychological well-being, freedom, general well-being, good health, and financially security. In reality, none of the caregivers had many of the characteristics they desired. The authors concluded that this study provided a new conceptualization of the term 'quality of life' and new insights into the personal meanings given to that term by this group of caregivers. However, it must be noted that the attributes they sought could be seen as ideal and frequently beyond reach, even in circumstances less dire than that of caring for a patient with Alzheimer's disease.

Caring for a person with dementia is a daunting task in and of itself. One aspect of caregiving that is not adequately addressed in the literature is the grief of the caregivers (spouses, children, and other intimates). Perhaps it is subsumed under the more common term depression. There are, however, fundamental differences in those two concepts. Grief is a normal human response to loss, and depression is a clinical state. The caregiver characteristics associated with dementia are not altogether unpredictable. The age, psychological state, pre-morbid health, and financial state of the caregiver have consequences for the quality of care that she/he is able to provide. Nevertheless, the emotional and health costs of caregiving are frequently high.

Finally, we present a summary of some of the research findings related to cultural differences as they influence caregiver responses in their performance of that role. We review three studies that tend to demonstrate more similarities than differences in caregivers from diverse cultures providing care for someone with dementia (Aguilia, Onor, Trevisiol, Negro, et al., 2004; Nomura, Inoue, Kamimura, Shimodera, et al., 2005; Pang, Chow, Cummings, Leung, et al., 2002; Salguero, Kohn, Salguero, & Marotta, 1998). However, there are also interesting differences.

In a comparative study of caregiver burden in Guatemala and Rhode Island, the authors found that the Guatemalans had less institutional care and more informal care compared to their counterparts in Rhode Island (Salguero, Kohn, Salguero, & Marotta, 1998). Guatemalans brought their patients earlier to the doctors upon the appearance of dementia-related symptoms and experienced poorer perceived burden than the Rhode Islanders. Aguglia and associates (2004) in their study of caregiver burden associated with AD in Italy concluded that the caregiver burden worsened as the disease progressed. There were also social and economic costs associated with caregiving. Deterioration in the health of the caregivers was associated with a reduction of independence in daily life of the patients and an increase in behavioural problems. The authors noted that parallels could be drawn between their findings and those involving the American caregivers. Pang and associates (2002) noted some difference in Chinese and American caregivers. They were surprised to find that American and Chinese caregivers exhibited similar distress or lack thereof in response to a variety of neuropsychiatric symptoms in the patients. Chinese caregivers, however, were less affected by depression and apathy in the Alzheimer's patients than were the American caregivers.

In short, while there are indeed some cultural differences in the caregiving of Alzheimer's patients, which may also be a factor of the availability of resources, such as a reliance on informal care, there are many similarities. Some of the differences are one of degree rather than substance. Nevertheless, it is important for clinicians to have some understanding of the cultural issues of their patients and caregivers, as they might have implications for the caregivers' health and well-being.

Summary

One fact to emerge with much clarity is that caring for a patient with dementia can and often does exact a heavy price. How taxing that might be is a function, among other factors, of the severity of the disease (presence of neuropsychiatric symptoms), the age of the caretaker (usually over 55 years), the caretaker's relationship with the patient (mostly a spouse), the availability of community resources, cultural factors, gender (usually female), and pre-existing medical condition(s) in the caregivers. Caring for a dementia patient is not just a challenge to the health of the caregiver; it can even hasten death. We also noted that depression or depressive symptoms are common in this population. In the following section we investigate the risk of developing clinical depression for the caregivers of patients with dementia.

Caregiver Depression

References were made in the preceding section to the relationship between caregiver stress and depression. In the following pages we explore in more depth the recent literature on some aspects, such as prevalence and risk factors, of caregiver depression. Even a cursory glance at this body of literature, which is substantial, reveals that depression in caregivers is almost ubiquitous. We shall presently review the predictors of depression in this population. We begin by reviewing two meta-analytic reports on the association between depression and caregiving (Black & Almeida, 2004; Pinquart & Sorensen, 2004). Second, we shall examine a few reports on large-scale studies that investigated this relationship (Clayburn, Stones, Hadjistavropoulos, & Tuokko, 2000; Covinsky, Newcomer, Fox, Wood, et al., 2003; O'Rourke, Cappeliez, & Neufeld, 2007; Schulz, McGinnis, Zhang, Martire, et al., 2008). Finally, the literature on predictors of depression in caregivers (Mahoney, Regan, Katona, & Livingston, 2005; Neundorfer, McClendon, Smyth, Strauss, & McCallum, 2006; Shua-Haim, Haim, Kuo, & Smith, 2001; Takahashi, Tanaka, & Miyaoka, 2005; Waite, Bebbington, Skelton-Robinson, & Orrell, 2004) shall be examined. Although the three aspects outlined above are interrelated, we have separated them for the convenience of reporting them.

The absence of epidemiological studies related to the incidence and prevalence of depression in the caregivers of dementia patients is truly conspicuous. However, there is one Canadian study that conducted a national epidemiologic study of dementia prevalence and the health and welfare of care providers (O'Rourke, Cappliez, & Neufeld, 2007). Patients and caregivers were assessed at three points over a ten-year period. Only family members who resided with the patients (n=96 pairs) were included in this study. The sample consisted of 37 men and 59 women with dementia. The caregivers consisted of adult children (51%), spouses (43.2%), and 2 sisters and 3 daughters-in-law. Depression in caregivers was measured by the twenty-item Center for Epidemiologic Studies depression (CES-D) scale at baseline and Time 2. A ten-item scale of CES-D was administered at Time 3. Caregivers' health status was also assessed at Times 1 and 2 by asking comprehensive questions about their health over preceding year. At Time 3 a brief health status survey was administered.

The result was unequivocal in its key finding that caregivers presenting with measurable depressive symptoms at multiple points (34.4%, 31.3%, and 26% at Times 1, 2, and 3) of measurement reported declining physical health over time. The health of all caregiver groups had declined at Time 3. The authors concluded that, in keeping with previous findings, depressive symptoms were associated with declining health at each point of measurement. The strength of this study was that participants were followed over a period of nearly ten years. Causal assertions were based on the longitudinal nature of this study and not simple correlational data.

Pinquart and Sorensen (2004), in a meta-analysis involving sixty studies, used the following criteria for inclusion in their analysis: (1) informal caregivers of older adults were assessed; (2) associations of caregiving stressors and uplifts with indications of subjective well-being were reported as correlations that could be converted to statistical measures; and (3) the studies were in English or German, or in a language for which the authors were able to obtain translation. About 20% of the literature surveyed was eliminated as it failed to meet the inclusion criteria. We report on two hypotheses of direct relevance to our topic that were tested in this meta-analysis.

The first hypothesis tested whether associations between caregiving stressors and uplifts with depression and subjective well-being would be domain-specific or whether cross-over effects could be observed. All measures of caregiving stressors were significantly related to caregiver depression, supporting the domain-specific effects hypothesis. In addition, a significant large negative correlation between caregiver depression and subjective well-being was found. The second hypothesis proposed that impairments of the patients would show stronger inverse relationships with subjective well-being than the intensity of caregiving. This expectation received much statistical support. Physical impairments and behavioural problems of the patient showed stronger associations with low subjective well-being than did the indicators of the intensity of caregiving. In short, uplifts of caregiving were associated with subjective well-being and caregiving stressors were associated with depression. Black and Almeida (2004), in their meta-analysis of thirty articles, supported previous findings that behavioural and psychological symptoms predicted burden of care and depression.

Clayburn and associates (2000) reported a study involving 613 patients with AD either at home or in institutions and their informal caregivers. One central finding of this study was the role of the appraisal of burden by the caregivers, which had significant impact on their sense of well-being. A higher frequency of disturbing behaviour, caring for a community-dwelling patient, and low levels of informal support were predictors of high levels of depression. More psychologically disturbed patients also received less help from family and friends.

In one of the largest cross-sectional studies conducted to analyse predictors of caregiver depression in caregivers of AD patients, Covinsky and colleagues (2003) confirmed very high rates of depression in the caregivers. Of 5627 patients, 32% had six or more symptoms of depression on the Geriatric Depression Scale-15. Independent patient predictors included being younger (65 years compared to 85 years); being White or Hispanic compared to Black; having less than a high school education; and behavioural disturbance (angry and aggressive patient).

Independent caregiver predictors of depression included a low income (less than $10,000 compared to $20,000 or more per year); the relationship to patient (wife compared to son of male patients); hours spent caregiving (40–79 hours compared to fewer than 40 hours); and functional dependence (Activities of Daily Living dependent compared to Instrumental Activities of Daily Living independent).

The authors concluded: 'We found that caregiver depression is a complex clinical and social problem, influenced, in part by the ethnicity of the patient, as well as multiple patient and caregiver characteristics. Like other common problems related to aging, caregiver depression is best approached by viewing it as a problem induced by the interactive effects of multiple risk factors, rather than a problem induced by a single dominant risk factor' (p. 1013).

The findings of another study (Schulz, McGinnis, Zhang, Martire, et al., 2008) that investigated the caregiver–depression relationship and use of the antidepressants complemented the findings of the above study. This was also a large-scale study involving 1222 dementia patients. The prevalence of two types of patient suffering, namely, emotional and existential distress, were explored. So was their independent relationship with caregiver depression and antidepressant medication use. Standardized instruments were used to assess a patient's cognitive function, suffering, memory problems, activities of daily living, and instrumental activities of daily living. Caregiver depression was assessed using the CES-D.

The average age of the caregivers was 62 years, most were females (81%), and just under half of them were spouses (48.2%). The patients' average age was 79 years and about 60% were female. Findings showed that both aspects of perceived patient suffering contributed to caregiver depression. However, only existential suffering accounted for antidepressant use. African Americans and Hispanics were less likely to use antidepressants than Whites, and caregiver spouses were less likely to use medications than non-spousal caregivers. The caregivers of female patients also used less medications. Anxiety was present in 63.4% and sadness and depression in 63.4% of caregivers. The authors noted that this was the first study to show in a large sample that perceived patient suffering independently contributed to family caregiver depression and medication use.

Three relatively recent studies that dealt with predictors of depression in caregivers reported similar and differing results (Mahoney et al., 2005; Shua-Haim, Haim, Kuo, & Smith, 2001; Waite, Bebbington, Skelton-Robinson, & Orrell, 2004). Waite and colleagues investigated 72 caregivers of patients with dementia. The inclusion criterion for the subjects was that they had to be over the age of 65. Most of the caregivers (84.7%) felt that the person with dementia was in control of their relationship, and another 56.9% had a confiding relationship with someone they saw daily. Live in caregivers were more depressed than non-live-in caregivers. Age, gender, and living arrangements influenced the risk for depression. In this population, 43.1% of the caregivers were depressed. Three factors that predicted depression in the caregivers were (1) lack of a confiding relationship; (2) depression in the person with dementia; and (3) living with a person with dementia.

Mahoney and colleagues (2005) reported depression in a much smaller proportion of the caregivers (10.5%). However, the risk factors for depression included (1) care recipient irritability; (2) caregivers reporting poor health; and (3) poor-quality relationship with care recipient. The subjects were 153 people with dementia and their caregivers. All 153 caregivers participated in the project. Depression was found in 38%

of the caregivers. Shua-Haim and associates (2001), in their investigation of risk factors for depression in caregivers, identified (1) depression in the dementia patient; (2) poor function in the activities of daily living; and (3) the presence of hallucination (neuropsychiatric symptoms).

Summary

Approximately one-third of caregivers of dementia patients develop depression. Major risk factors that predict depression in the caregivers are depression in the patient with dementia, the presence of neuropsychiatric symptoms, the quality of the relationship of the caregiver with the care recipient, the level of impairment in the patient, female caregivers, and caregiver health. Caregiving for a person with dementia undoubtedly carries health and psychological risks for the caregivers. The question we address below is how that might influence the social support role of the caregivers of persons with dementia.

Social Support

The significance of caregiver support for improved health outcomes cannot be overstated. As the following review will show, empirical studies have demonstrated a positive relationship between caregiver support and a better health outcome for patients with dementia. Yet, caregivers of dementia patients are a relatively high-risk group for morbidity or even mortality. Empirical evidence for their vulnerability to psychiatric disorders, especially depression, is considerable. Roughly 30% of intimate caregivers usually develop depression. In addition, many of the caregivers are elderly and have ongoing health issues. All these factors compromise the ability of the caregivers to provide support that may have some protective or buffering effects. In fact, an extensive literature search failed to produce much related to the buffering effect of spousal or family-member social support for dementia patients. On the other hand, there exists a plethora of research that shows that when caregivers and patients with dementia are involved in formal programs for coping with dementia, the caregivers do fulfil a supportive role for the patients. This body of literature is truly diverse, reporting wide-ranging intervention programs to help support the caregivers of dementia patients. We present a brief summary of some of that literature.

The effectiveness of caregiver support, albeit somewhat indirectly, is reported by a few studies. Droes, Meiland, Schmitz, and van Tilburg (2005) reported a study with 112 dementia patients who visited a number of day care facilities in Amsterdam. Patients in the experimental group (n=89) received support from the Meeting Center Support Program as well as from their caregivers. Patients in the control group (n=23) received day care only. After seven months, results showed that patients and caregivers in the experimental group compared to regular day care did significantly better in the domain of behaviour problems, mood, and depression. The conclusion was that the Meeting Center Support Program proved to be more effective than regular day care. Another point of note was that providing support for caregivers enhanced their effectiveness in their support role.

A systematic review with a meta-analysis was conducted to estimate the overall effectiveness of non-medical support programs for caregivers and patients with dementia that were intended to delay institutionalization (Spijker, Vernooij-Dassen, Vasse, Adang, et al., (2008). Thirteen support programs with 9043 patients were included in this meta-analysis. The estimated overall effectiveness showed that these programs significantly decreased the odds of institutionalization. Furthermore, actively involving caregivers in making choices about treatments distinguished effective from non-effective programs. The benefits of caregiver support for dementia patients was confirmed. This review furnished powerful data to show the benefits of involving caregivers in support programs.

A recent study (Fortinsky, Kolldorft, Kleppinger, & Kenyon-Pesce, 2009) found only qualified support for the key finding (delayed institutionalization for dementia patients) of the above review. The main objective of this study was to examine the efficacy of an individualized dementia care consultation intervention for family caregivers of patients with dementia. Consultation was provided by the dementia care consultants based at an Alzheimer's association chapter in Hartford, Connecticut. The caregivers in the intervention group received individualized counselling and support over a twelve-month period, and the care plans developed with family caregivers including the referring family physicians. The subjects in the control group only received information on community and educational resources, but no care consultation. A total of 84 caregivers participated.

The intervention failed to reach a statistically lower rate of nursing home admissions of caregivers' relatives with dementia. Nevertheless, the trend was favourable to the intervention group compared to the control group. The results showed only modest benefits accruing from care consultation intervention in the objective of keeping the care recipients at home. The majority of the caregivers did not discuss the care plans with their physicians. The authors noted that there were many barriers to maintaining an ongoing dialogue and collaboration between primary care physicians and a voluntary sector such as an Alzheimer's association chapter. This program was, at best, nominally successful.

This section concludes with a report that, in fact, demonstrated the role of social support with dementia patients. This Dutch study (de Vugt, Stevens, Aalten, & Verhey, 2005) proposed to explore caregiver management strategies on the functioning of dementia patients. Ninety-nine patients with dementia and their caregivers were followed up for a year. Three management strategies employed by the caregivers were identified, based on the level of acceptance of the situation of the dementia-related problems. Non-accepting caregivers were categorized as 'non-adapters'; caregiver acceptance was divided into two categories, nurturers and supporters.

Non-adapters reported significantly more hyperactivity symptoms in patients and felt less competent than the 'supporters.' Supporters were the most competent and reported the fewest hyperactivity symptoms in their patients. The authors concluded that caregiver management strategies seemed to be associated with behavioural problems in dementia patients and the degree to which the caregivers felt competent to deal with the situation(s). Teaching caregivers management strategies might enhance their ability to deal more effectively with behavioural problems associated with dementia.

Summary

First and foremost, there seems to be overwhelming evidence to support the value of programs designed to help the caregiver of dementia patients. As noted earlier, that body of literature is vast. We have barely scratched its surface here. Nevertheless, we offer an overview to show the necessity of providing training and support programs for a rather vulnerable group who often suffer negative health consequences due to the burden of care. We also note that delaying institutionalization as a consequence of effective social support may be considered a harsh outcome measure. Goals such as a reduction in behavioural problems or enhancing of functional levels could also serve as worthwhile outcome measures. One last point of note is that the buffering effect of social support in the context of dementia patients remains an under-researched area. The reasons for that are not hard to surmise. Behavioural combined with neuropsychiatric problems are endemic to this population. Caring for them poses a kind of challenge that is often hazardous.

Conclusion

Dementia is a disease mostly of old age with serious medical and social repercussions. As our society ages, the number of people afflicted with dementia will continue to rise. The question of social support for this population is complex. In fact, the general notion of the positive outcome of social support has limited relevance to dementia. The nature of the support and care that patients with dementia require has telling consequences for those who provide such care. First and foremost, not infrequently the caregivers of the dementia patients, especially spouses, who tend to be older, are confronted with old age themselves. The caregiver's health is frequently a victim of the burden of caregiving associated with dementia. As we noted, the dementia patients suffer from many neuropsychological symptoms. In advanced stages of the disease they need constant supervision, as they may wander away or engage in inappropriate or even dangerous behaviour. That accounts for the very heavy burden associated with caregiving for dementia patients.

The health and social cost for the caregivers is significant. Almost all the studies reveal that a full one-third of spouse/children caregivers develop depression. Anxiety is another common problem. The general morbidity level in these caregivers is also high. A few studies have even found an association between the caregiving of dementia patients and mortality. Social support for the caregivers has been demonstrated in study after study to be highly beneficial, not only for the caregivers, but also for the patients. We presented a limited review of that vast literature. Noteworthy is the fact that unlike the benefits of social support as observed in the preceding chapters, which generally protects the patient, this concept is turned upside down in relation to dementia. The need for social support is paramount for the caregivers of the dementia patient. Without the benefit of organized programs to support these caregivers, their existence can and does become precarious.

REFERENCES

Agulia, E., Onor, M., Trevisiol, M., Negro, C., et al. (2009). Stress in the caregivers of Alzheimer's patients: An experimental investigation in Italy. *Am. J.
Alzheimer's Disease and Other Dementias, 19,* 248–252.

Allegri, R., Sarasola, D., Serrano, C., Taragano, F., et al. (2006). Neuropsychiatric symptoms as a predictor of caregiver burden in Alzheimer's disease.
Neuropsychiatric Disease and Treatment, 2, 105–110.

Alzheimer's Association (2009). 2009 Alzheimer's disease facts and figures.
Alzheimer's Dementia, 5, 234–270.

Black, W., & Almeida, O. (2004). A systematic review of the association
between the behavioral and psychological symptoms of dementia and burden of care. *International Psychogeriatric, 16,* 295–315.

Clayburn, L., Stones, M., Hadjistavropoulos, T., & Tuokko, H. (2000). Predicting caregiver burden and depression in Alzheimer's disease. *J. Gerontol B
Psychol Sci Soc Sci., 55,* S2–13.

Covinsky, K., Newcomer, R., Fox, P., Wood, J., et al. (2003). Patient and caregiver characteristics associated with depression in caregivers of patients
with dementia. *Journal of General Internal Medicine, 18,*1006–1014.

de Vugt, M., Stevens, F., Aalten, P., & Verhey, F. (2005). Do [sic] looking after
family members influence behaviors of dementia patients. *Tijdschrift inst
voor en Geriatrie, 36,* 11–18.

Droes, R., Meiland, F., Schmitz, F., & van Tilburg, W. (2005). Effect of combined support for people with dementia and carers versus regular day
care on behavior and mood of persons with dementia: Results from multi-
center implementation study. *Tijdschrift voor Gerontologie en Geriatrie, 36,*
60–71.

Fortinsky, R., Kulldorft, M., Kleppinger, A., & Kenyon-Pesce, L. (2009).
Dementia care consultation for family caregivers: Collaborative model link-
ing an Alzheimer's association chapter with primary care physicians. *Aging
& Mental Health, 13,* 162–170.

Hebert, L., Scherr, P., Bienias, J., et al. (2003). Alzheimer disease in the US
population: Prevalence estimates using the 2000 census. *Arch. Neurol., 60,*
1119–1112.

Lindsay, J., Sykes, E., McDowell, I., Verreault, R., & Laurin, D. (2004). More
than epidemiology of Alzheimer's disease: Contributions of the Canadian
Study of Health and Aging. *Can. J. Psychiatry, 49,* 83–91.

Mahoney, R., Regan, C., Katona, C., & Livingston, G. (2005). Anxiety and
depression in family caregivers of people with Alzheimer's disease: The
Lased-Ad study. *Am. J. Geriatric Psychiat., 13,* 795–801.

Mausbach, B., von Kanel, R., Aschbacher, K., Roepke, S., et al. (2007). Spousal caregivers of patients with Alzheimer's disease show longitudinal increases in plasma levels of tissue-type plasminogen activator antigen. *Psychosomatic Medicine, 69*, 816–822.

Mitrani, V., Lewis, J., Feaster, D., Czaja, S., et al. (2006). The role of family functioning in the stress process of dementia caregivers: A structural family framework. *The Gerontologist, 46*, 97–105.

Neundorfer, M., McClendon, M., Smyth, K., Strauss, M., & McCallum, T. (2006). Does depression prior to caregiving increase vulnerability to depressive symptoms among caregivers of persons with Alzheimer's disease? *Aging & Mental Health, 10*, 606–615.

Nomura, H., Inoue, S., Kamimura, N., Shimodera, S., et al. (2005). A cross-cultural study on expressed emotion in carers of people with dementia and schizophrenia: Japan and England. *Social Psychiatry & Psychiatric Epidemiology, 40*, 564–570.

O'Rourke, N., Cappeliez, P., & Neufeld, E. (2007). Recurrent depressive symptomatology and physical health: A 10-year study of informal caregivers of persons with dementia. *Can. J. Psychiatry, 52*, 434–441.

Pang, F., Chow, T., Cummings, V., Leung, V., et al. (2002). Effects of neuropsychiatric symptoms of Alzheimer's disease on Chinese and American caregivers. *International J. Geriatric Psychiatry, 17*, 29–34.

Pinquart, M., & Sorensen, S. (2004). Association of caregiver stressors with subjective well-being and depressive mood: A meta-analytic comparison. *Aging and Mental Health, 8*, 438–449.

Plassman, K., Langa, K., Fisher, G., Heeringa, S., et al. (2007). Prevalence of dementia in the United States: The aging, demographics, and memory study. *Neuroepidemiology, 29*, 125–132.

Quinn, C., Clare, L., & Woods, B. (2009). The impact of the quality of relationship on the experiences and well-being of caregivers of people with dementia: A systematic review. *Aging and Mental Health, 13*, 143–154.

Salguero, R., Kohn, R., Salguero, L., & Marotta, C. (1998). Caregivers of persons with Alzheimer's disease: Cultural differences in perceived caregiver burden in Guatemala & Rhode Island. *J. Cross Cultural Gerontology, 13*, 229–240.

Sawa, G., Zaccai, J., Matthews, F., Davidson, J., et al. (2009). Prevalence, correlates and course of behavioral and psychological symptoms of dementia in population. *Br. J. Psychiatry, 194*, 212–219.

Schulz, R., & Beach, S. (1999). Caregiving as a risk factor for mortality: The caregiver health effects study. *JAMA, 282*, 2215–2219.

Schulz, R., McGinnis, K., Zhang, S., Martire, L., et al. (2008). Dementia patient suffering and caregiver depression. *Alzheimer's Disease & Associated Disorders, 22,* 170–176.

Serrano-Aguliar, P., Lopez-Batisda, J., & Yanes-Lopez, V. (2006). Impact on health-related quality of life and perceived burden of informal caregivers of individuals with Alzheimer's disease. *Neuroepidemiology, 27,* 136–142.

Shua-Haim, J., Haim, T., Shi, Y., Kuo, Y., & Smith, J. (2001). Depression among Alzheimer's caregivers: Identifying risk factors. *Am.J. Alzheimer's Disease and Other Dementias, 16,* 353–359.

Sink, K., Covinsky, K., Barnes, D., Newcomer, R., & Yaffe, K. (2006). Caregiver characteristics are associated with neuropsychiatric symptoms of dementia. *J. American Geriatric Society, 54,* 796–803.

Spijker, A., Vernooij-Dassen, M., Vasse, E., Adang, E., et al. (2008). Effectiveness of non-pharmacological interventions in delaying the institutionalization of patients with dementia. *J. Am. Geriatric Society, 56,* 1116–1128.

Takahashi, M., Tanaka, K., & Miyaoka, H. (2005). Depression and associated factors of informal caregivers versus professional caregivers of demented patients. *Psychiatry and Clinical Neurosciences, 59,* 473–480.

Van Den Wijngaart, M., Vernooij-Dassen, M., & Felling, A. (2007). The influence of stressors, appraisals and personal condition on the burden of spousal caregivers of persons with dementia. *Aging & Mental Health, 11,* 626–636.

Vellone, E., Piras, G., Talucci, C., & Cohen, M. (2007). Quality of life for caregivers of people with Alzheimer's disease. *J. Advanced Nursing, 61,* 222–231.

Vitaliano, P., Zhang, J., & Scanlan, J. (2003). Is caregiving hazardous to one's physical health? A meta-analysis. *Psychological Bulletin, 129,* 946–972.

Waite, A., Bebbington, P., Skelton-Robinson, M., & Orrell, M. (2004). Social factors and depression in carers of people with dementia. *International J. Geriatric psychiatry, 19,* 582–5.

7 Breast Cancer and Social Support: Special Challenges

The diagnosis of cancer almost always is an extremely anxiety-provoking event for the patient and intimates. For historical reasons this diagnosis is equated with a death sentence. While the survival rate for many cancers have risen significantly over the years, the initial response of fear and apprehension is almost universal. As our review will show, the prevalence of general distress and anxiety and depression for the patient and often family members is far from uncommon. We have chosen breast cancer for our purposes here.

Breast cancer is the most common form of cancer in women. The risk of cancer rises with age. Young women tend to have a low risk of breast cancer. However, cancer in young women tends to be larger and of a higher grade with poorer prognosis, resulting in a higher risk of recurrence and death from breast cancer when compared to older women (Yankaskas, 2006). Yankaskas reported a European study showing cancer data for adolescents (aged 15–19) versus young adults (20–24 years) that found survival worse for the adolescents. The five-year survival rate for these very young women was 67.5%. A Swiss study showed that five-year breast cancer survival rates for women aged 35 or younger was 92% compared to 90% for women 36–45 years.

A recent report on cancer prevalence in Canada showed that 'nearly 40% of ten-year prevalent cancer cases were either breast cancer (20.5%) or prostate (18.7%)' (Ellison and Wilkins, 2009). Breast cancer was also found to be dominant in the 40–49 years age group. The prevalence of breast cancer rose with age. Between the ages of 40 and 49, some 18,000 persons in Canada had breast cancer. This number rises to over 20,000 for those aged 80 years and over. It was also noted that breast cancer was most prevalent, along with prostate cancer, partly due to high incidence, but also because of the improved rate of survival. The authors noted that while in Canada the number of newly diagnosed cases of cancer continue to rise, so does the rate of survival. In the United States the five-year survival rate beyond diagnosis for breast cancer is estimated to be 89% (American Cancer Society, 2007).

Breast Cancer and Emotional Distress

A sweeping review of the epidemiologic literature on major depression in breast cancer patients (Finn, Thomas-Rich, Katon, Cowley, et al., 2008) noted that breast cancer patients are most vulnerable for depression during the first year of diagnosis. A diagnosis of breast cancer is associated with considerable stress for the patients. Finn and colleagues found that while there was extensive research to find confirmation for that fact, few studies investigated the epidemiology and treatment of major depression in breast cancer patients.

Major depression in patients with breast cancer, caregiver burden, and distress are often major issues for families (Grunfeld, Coyle, Whelan, Clinch, et al., 2004; Wagner, Bigatti, & Storniolo, 2006). We shall presently consider the issue of caregiver distress and other relationship problems. As for the prevalence of major depression in patients with breast cancer, Finn and colleagues (2008) concluded that determining the actual prevalence of major depression in this population was problematic largely due to a multitude of methodological problems in the studies they reviewed. They estimated that the prevalence of major depression was around 10–25%. One of their telling findings was that 'the depression rate for breast cancer appears to be higher than most other cancers with the exception of pancreatic and oropharyngeal cancers' (p. 119).

Apart from major depression, many of these patients encounter a variety of psychosocial issues that impinge on their general well-being and had consequences for their intimates. One rather unusual study examined the role of personal control after breast surgery (Henselmans, Sanderman, Bass, Smink, & Ranchor, 2009). Loss of control when confronted with a diagnosis such as breast cancer could be considered a predictable feeling. This longitudinal study was designed to gain insight into the changes that might occur due to a breast cancer diagnosis in personal control and the stress-buffering effect of personal control. Personal control was assessed with the seven-item Master List in breast cancer patients: (1) not treated with chemotherapy (n=47); (2) breast cancer patients treated with chemotherapy (n=32); and (3) in healthy women (n=58) at 3, 9, and 15 months after diagnosis.

The results showed that patients treated with chemotherapy, and who faced a longer period in treatment and with poorer prognosis, reported lower levels of personal control than the healthy subjects. Three months post-diagnosis predicted a lessening of distress only in patients treated with chemotherapy. Surprisingly, women treated with chemotherapy seemed to have a higher sense of control over life than the healthy subjects at nine months post-diagnosis. The stress-buffering hypothesis received only modest support for its effect on control. One main and somewhat surprising conclusion of this study was that it was not the breast cancer diagnosis, but the necessary treatment modality and prognosis that defined the stress experience. There was no explanation given for the relative absence of the feelings of loss of control at the point of diagnosis. After nine months, at the termination of treatment, patients were no longer monitored closely, and were expected to resume their normal life. There was time to reflect, and the thought of recurrence made it hard to preserve a sense of control. Maintaining a sense of control was hardest in this group during this period. Personal control was a valuable resource, but threatened when confronted with an unknown future.

Psychosocial problems ranging from concerns regarding body image to sexual concerns to lower quality of life due to medical treatment are relatively common (Avis, Crawford, & Manuel, 2004; Baucom, Porter, Kirby, Gremore, & Keefe, 2006). Avis and colleagues surveyed psychosocial problems in 204 women between the ages of 25 and 50 years diagnosed with breast cancer. The mean age at diagnosis was 42 years. Forty patients had mastectomy with no reconstruction and another 47 patients had mastectomy and subsequent reconstruction. The sample was primarily Caucasian (96%). Most were married (82%). The authors used the Cancer Rehabilitation Evaluation System (CARES) and open-ended questions for data collection.

The authors closely examined individual items on CARES where 40% or more expressed concerns. They were: uncomfortable about changes in their body (46%); difficulty getting lubricated during sex (40.7%); lack of interest in sex (41.7%). For some the following problems were relevant: worry about early onset of menopause (57.3%); pregnancy affecting breast cancer (48.3%); ability to get pregnant (41.1%). Answers to the open-ended questions confirmed the empirical findings. Concerns about weight gain, hair loss, feeling disfigured or lop-sided, relationship with partners, and job-related concerns such as fear of losing employment due to tiredness or simply quitting work were reported by many of the subjects. This study confirmed that many, if not most, of the psychosocial problems relate to the insult to their sense of identity experienced by these women. This may have a profound effect on the partner relationship. Many of the findings of this study were noted in a major review of the psychosocial problems encountered by younger breast cancer survivors.

A comprehensive review of the literature on psychosocial issues confronted by young women with breast cancer confirmed the findings of the preceding study (Baucom, Porter, Kirby, Gremore, and Keefe, 2006). This review is divided into two parts. The first part examines the psychosocial problems encountered by women with breast cancer, and the second is a review of interventions. Our focus is on the first section. Authors report on the symptoms and treatment side-effects, body image, and sexual functioning. Quality-of-life issues are also reported. Based on numerous investigations, young women compared to their older counterparts with breast cancer experience greater deterioration in their quality of life.

Women with breast cancer experience a wide range of physical symptoms not only during treatment, but after as well, including menopause, infertility, menstrual changes, lymphedema, and pain. Many experience physical limitations with physical and recreational activities. Younger women are confronted with the possibility of never having children. Hence, it is not at all surprising that younger women experience significant deterioration in their quality of life compared to older women.

Almost two-thirds of women with breast cancer express unhappiness with their body image. The reviewers noted: 'Given the surgical procedures for breast cancer remove a part of the body and typically alter a woman's physical appearance in an area that is given great value in Western societies, it is understandable that women with breast cancer often present concerns regarding body image' (p. 105). Concern about body image was predictably most frequent in patients who had a mastectomy alone, followed by women with a mastectomy who had reconstruction, followed by patients who had a lumpectomy. Many of these women experience what amounts to rapid aging of their bodies with regard to skin and bone density.

Given a sense of having to live with an imperfect body, many young women with breast cancer experience sexual difficulties. According to this review some one-third of women reported dissatisfaction with their sexual life. Younger women, in particular, were most vulnerable for experiencing sexual problems. These sexual difficulties seemed to persist for as much as ten years following diagnosis. The problems consisted of infrequent sexual activities, vaginal dryness, and reduced breast sensitivity. Treatments of breast cancer which include chemo-therapy, radiation therapy, and surgery all tend to impact negatively on the sexuality of these women.

Summary

Breast cancer in young women, in particular, presents serious chal-lenges. Major depression, distorted body image, deterioration in their quality of life, and dissatisfaction with their sexual activities are not uncommon in this population. In fact, when the risk for depression is combined with all the other problems, it would appear that a significant proportion of these young women confront many, if not all, of these problems. They are essentially interrelated. In the section that follows, we examine the impact of breast cancer on the partner relationship.

What Happens to Partners?

The essence of the main finding for the spouse or caregiver is that the level of distress expressed by the breast cancer patient is mirrored by the caregiver (Hodges, Humphries, & MacFarlane, 2005). This was the central conclusion of a meta-analysis of the research literature on the stress of caregivers of cancer patients (ibid.). Their analysis was based on 21 studies that met the pre-defined inclusion criteria. The analy-sis was based on 1098 dyads. Based on a standard statistical method employed in meta-analysis, the authors noted that there was a signifi-cant positive relationship between patient and caregiver self-reported psychological distress. The effect size established by this analysis was also robust. The mutuality between the caregiver and patient distress – that is, when one partner becomes distressed, it is more than likely that the other partner will also be – is telling. However, reasons behind the reciprocal nature of the response to stress are not well understood, and the authors noted that this phenomenon was yet to be researched. They also reported that there existed a sub-group of patients and caregivers who were at higher risk of suffering from psychological distress. It should be noted that this study was based on cancer and not exclusively breast cancer patients.

This central finding of mutuality of distress in cancer patients and their partners was also confirmed in a study of couples dealing with breast and prostate cancer (Kim, Kashy, Wellisch, Spillers, et al., 2008). A total of 168 married cancer-survivor caregiver dyads participating in the American Cancer Society's Study of Cancer-Survivors-1 and Quality of Life Survey for Caregivers completed the required questionnaires for this study. Cancer patients were diagnosed with breast or prostate cancer approximately two years before their participation in the study. The participants were middle-aged, Caucasian, relatively educated, and affluent. Contrary to expectation, prostate cancer survivors reported better physical health than their caregivers.

However, there was evidence that in both types of cancer, partners were similar in their levels of psychological distress. Older prostate cancer survivors reported better mental health. As for physical health, both survivors and caregivers revealed that more psychologically distressed individuals had poorer physical health. One telling conclusion of this study was that two years from the time of diagnosis, the study participants displayed normal levels of psychological well-being and quality of life. Finally, the authors noted that their findings showed that when a couple was dealing with as serious an illness as cancer, the extent to which women psychologically adjust to the situation played a key role not only in their own well-being, but also in that of their partners.

Brusilovskiy, Mitstifer, and Salzer (2009) conducted a study to explore the relationship between a woman's perception of her partner's emotional, behavioural, and intimate adaptation to her breast cancer. Sixty-six subjects participated. Of these 59 were married, 97% were white, 92% had education beyond high school, and 94% were receiving treatment for the first time. Partner adaptation was measured by using three open-ended questions. Appropriate instruments were used to measure distress, well-being, and social support.

Results showed that women whose partners' intimate adaptation was positive had significantly lower distress. 85% of the participants (47/55) reported their partners' behavioural adaptation to be positive. Women who perceived their partners' adaptation as positive were likely to report better quality of life, self-efficacy, hope, and social support. Statistically, this study demonstrated that there was an association between the overall view of a partner's adaptation and a woman's distress, well-being, and social support.

Shands, Lewis, Sinsheimer, and Cochrane (2006) reported a study involving 29 women with breast cancer and their partners. These couples were engaged in a 'coaching' program to deal with their illness-related concerns. The average length of time since the diagnosis for the patients was 5.7 months. Eleven of these women had lumpectomies and another 28 had mastectomies. Their average age was 41 years. The average length of relationship was 15 years and the number of children living at home ranged from 0–3 (median 2). The ages of the children ranged from birth to 21 years (mean of 9 years).

Data obtained for this study was based on extensive audio-taped interviews. Analysis yielded 12 categories of concerns that could be divided into four main domains. These domains and the problems under them were:

1 Dealing with tension in the relationship;
   Not knowing how to respond to her;
   Wanting him to understand;
   Needing to know what it is like to touch.
2 Needing to be together as a couple;
   Needing time without the children;
   Needing to do more fun things,
   Tired of listening to her worries.
3 Wondering about the children;
   Trying to read the impact;
   Worrying about the lingering effects;
   Not knowing how to respond.
4 Managing the threat of breast cancer;
   Preventing a recurrence;
   Fearing a recurrence;
   Needing assistance in seeking medical information.

This descriptive study provided a portrait of problems experienced by cancer patients and their partners. From a clinical perspective, this kind of information is invaluable. These results supported the proposition that the first year of living with and adjusting to breast cancer can have a profound impact on the entire family's well-being. An important conclusion to emerge from this study was that the couples, instead of avoiding the relationship issues that confronted them, were willing to deal with them.

Skerrett (1998) conducted a qualitative study involving 20 patients with breast cancer and their partners. They ranged in age from 34 to 73 years. It was the first marriage for 18 couples. Twelve patients had lumpectomies, five had modified radical mastectomies, and three had radical mastectomies. Altogether 20 couples were interviewed 18 to 31 months after diagnosis. They engaged in semi-structured interviews as couples and individually about their communication patterns, beliefs regarding illness and health, problem-solving techniques, feelings of loss and disfigurement, and topics relevant to their experience. These interviews were audio-taped and coded using Grounded Theory, which enabled the investigator to code and categorize the data.

It is noteworthy that the majority of the subjects were from a support group, and by definition they were able to seek help. In short, this was a highly selected group. The overall functioning of the couples was satisfactory. The level of distress was low, and as a group they seemed to be mastering the challenges of living with the disease. The characteristics of the couples by cluster were as follows:

High Adapters (85%):	At Risk (15%):
Challenging impact;	Devastating impact;
United coping philosophy;	Lack of mutuality;
Effective communication;	Strained communication;
Effective use of multi-generational legacies;	Problem in using such legacies;
Articulated beliefs;	Absent or conflictual beliefs;
Resilient sexually	Multiple stressors (medical complications, past losses)

One interesting finding was that the longer-married couples were among the more resilient. The author speculated that living together for a substantial period strengthened mutuality and promoted positive attitudes. The younger couples reported a stronger sense of shock, fear, and a sense of loss of control following diagnosis. These couples felt guarded about their future together, fearing future losses. Parents with young children were also anxious about their ability to raise them into their adulthood. This qualitative study was included as it provided details about the relationships, delving into their hopes and fears. Overall, the study was able to show, with all the limitations of a selected sample, that breast cancer patients and their partners do manage to deal with the fallout of the disease effectively. But some do not and they must be identified and treated.

So far all the studies we have reported were designed to investigate multiple problems encountered by breast cancer patients and their partners. Our next study (Manne, Ostroff, Norton, Fox, et al., 2006) is a departure to the extent that it examines the types communication that breast cancer couples employ. This longitudinal study involved 147 patients with early-stage breast cancer and 127 partners, and investigated their communication patterns during and after breast cancer treatment.

The instrument used to assess patterns of communication was the Communications Pattern Questionnaire (CPQ), which was adapted for cancer patients. Other instruments were used to assess marital quality and functional impairment in the patients only. Three sub-scales of CPQ, mutual constructive communication, demand-withdraw communication, and mutual avoidance, were investigated.

Relationship dissatisfaction reported by patients and partners was very low and did not change over time. Cancer-related relationship communication did not change significantly for either patient or partner. All three communication patterns were significant predictors of patient distress at Time 2. Patients reporting more mutually constructive communication predictably had lower levels of distress. Mutual constructive communication was associated with lower distress among patients regardless of their levels of physical impairment.

All three communication variables were significant predictors of partner distress at Time 2. Mutual constructive communication and demand-withdraw communication were associated with relationship satisfaction, but Mutual Avoidance was not at Time 2.

This study had five key findings:

1 Patient and partner distress and relationship satisfaction were a function of their perceptions of how they communicated about the cancer-related stressors they faced;
2 Physical impairment influenced the associations between constructive communication and patient distress;
3 Cancer-related communication did not change over the nine-month study period;
4 Couples were at variance in their perceptions of communication with each other; and

5 A patient's perception of communication affected her partner's
   distress and marital satisfaction, but the reverse was not true.

The authors pointed out the necessity of understanding the clinical significance of communication patterns and styles between cancer
patients and their partners, and the need for couple-focused intervention. This type of intervention might help in reducing the avoidance of
discussion of cancer-related stressors, and work at enhancing constructive communication.

Our next three studies are concerned with the reactions and adjustment of partners of breast cancer patients (Dorval, Guay, Mondor,
Masse, et al., 2005; Feldman & Broussard, 2006; Hoga, Mello, & Dias,
2008). Hoga and associates, in a Brazilian study, reported on the
response of 17 partners of breast cancer patients. These interviews were
conducted post-mastectomy, but the patients were still involved in
receiving hospital outpatient care. All 17 patients had a mastectomy: 11
had total unilateral, 2 total bilateral, and 4 modified radical unilateral.
Patients' ages ranged from 53 to 84 years, the length of relationship
from 21 to 50 years. This was a qualitative study. In-depth interviews
were conducted with all the male partners.

Five main themes emerged from the analysis of the narratives. They
were:

1 Initial reaction to the diagnosis: A husband's initial reaction to the
   diagnosis was in some ways predictable. They were collectively
   angry, nervous, annoyed, sad, and even depressed. Many experienced despair. The thought of losing their partner provoked a strong
   emotional reaction.
2 Involvement in caregiving: All the husbands were involved as the
   primary caregivers. The authors noted that this involved psychological support, attending all treatments in hospitals, and helping with
   daily care, such as bathing, changing, and so on.
3 Social support received: Breast cancer had a profound impact on
   family dynamics and the roles of family members. All members
   were asked to contribute to caring for the patient. In addition,
   neighbours and friends were also very supportive during the entire
   length of the patients' illness.
4 Effects of cancer on the couples' relationship: The mastectomy did
   not have any major effect on the marital relationship. Preservation
   of life was their main priority at that stage. Breast cancer was seen

by the partners as a life-threatening disease and they were entirely focused on providing support to their sick partners. Nor was their intimate relationship significantly altered. One critical observation was that due to the age of the subjects sex was not central to the relationship.

5 Evaluation of care provided by the institution: In the main, all partners were satisfied with the care patients received. They had confidence in the staff, the administrative organization, and the technical resources available for treatment.

Several points are noteworthy. First is the age of the couples, ranging from early fifty to the middle eighties. These were individuals in long-term relationships, which might suggest a relationship predicated on mutuality. The sexual aspect of the relationship or the issues related to body image for the patients were less critical than they would have been with a younger group of women who had a mastectomy. The reaction of the partners to the diagnosis of breast cancer had a universal quality. Their willingness and ability to provide support and also mobilize other forms of social support is noteworthy. At the end, the strength of these relationships accounted for much of the findings reported by this study.

Feldman and Broussard (2006) reported on 71 male partners of newly diagnosed breast cancer patients. The mean age of the men was 51 years. The average length of relationship (either married or partnered) was 19.9 years. The population was well educated, and 61% of the households reported an annual income of $90,000 or more.

Two hypothesis were tested:

1 Male partners of breast cancer patients who report higher levels of positive dyadic coping strategies will report higher levels of adjustment; and
2 Male partners of breast cancer patients who report higher levels of negative dyadic coping strategies will report lower levels of adjustment.

The Quality of Life Spouses Scale was used to assess emotional well-being, and illness intrusiveness was measured by Illness Intrusiveness Rating Scale. Dyadic coping was measured by the Dyadic Coping Scale.

The results were mixed. Multivariate analysis was conducted to test the two hypotheses. Hypothesis 1 failed to achieve statistically significant findings for predicting either emotional well-being or illness intrusiveness based on the results of six regression models. Hypothesis 2 also failed to support hostile dyadic coping and the avoidance of dyadic coping levels as predictors of the men's emotional well-being.

Data from the bivariate analysis showed that longer relationships were associated with less illness intrusiveness, a lower rate of depression, and higher rates of partners' emotional well-being. Men who were treated for depression before the onset of the breast cancer diagnosis reported lower emotional adjustment and more illness intrusiveness and employed fewer effective coping strategies.

This study yielded mixed results. The two main hypotheses were not supported by the data. On the other hand, higher levels of hostile dyadic patterns predicted poorer adjustment with illness adjustment. Men with a history of depression had difficulty in adapting to their partners' illness. There was some evidence that the partners' illness had negative consequences for work, sleep, the sexual relationship, and the relationship with other family members. The necessity of working with couples experiencing breast cancer was noted.

Our final study (Dorval, Guay, Mondor, Masse, et al., 2005) investigated the factors that brought breast cancer patients and their partners closer. The sample consisted of 282 couples. The women were newly diagnosed with non-metastatic breast cancer. Most of the patients (84%) had a partial mastectomy. Their ages ranged between 28 and 78 years. Most of the couples had lived together between 15 and 56 years. Information about the effects of the disease and its treatment on the closeness of their relationship was obtained at the twelve-month interview using a single question.

The results showed that 42% of the 282 couples reported that breast cancer had a positive impact on the relationship in terms of promoting closeness. Four factors accounted for the increase in closeness:

1   spouse reporting the patient as confidant;
2   spouse getting advice from the patient in the first two weeks about coping with breast cancer;
3   patients reporting more affection from their partners three months from the point of diagnosis; and
4   spouse accompanying her to the surgery.

A simple question was asked to elicit data. This was a longitudinal study, one of its kind, that attempted to isolate those characteristics that might predict a promotion of closeness between partners following a diagnosis of non-metastatic cancer. This study confirmed findings from previous studies that partners who support each other in a reciprocal manner early after breast cancer diagnosis each individually were inclined to be more satisfied with their relationship.

Summary

In sum, partner-related issues are many and varied in relation to breast cancer. On the other hand, long-term relationships appear to be less problematic and more supportive. More distress in the patient is also predictive of more distress in the partner. Many partners of breast cancer patients are also susceptible for a high degree of distress. Our last study reported that 42% of the partners of breast cancer patients experienced an improved relationship following the diagnosis of breast cancer. This also suggests that 58% did not. There was some evidence that those couples who were in support groups reported less stress in their relationships. Overall, almost all the studies emphasized the importance of some kind of support/intervention program for the breast cancer patient and her partner.

Social Support and Breast Cancer

The critical question is, Does social support, especially spousal support, confirm the buffering hypothesis? We acknowledge that, beside spousal/partner support, other kinds of support, such as peer support groups, are important in any consideration of social support for breast cancer patients. However, given the centrality and significance of the partner relationship with this population, we confine our review to the effectiveness of the spousal/partner relationship. We begin by reporting on two major reviews. The first is a meta-analytic review on the influence of social network on cancer mortality (Pinquart & Duberstein, 2009) and the second is a systematic review of the literature on the influence of psychosocial factors on breast cancer (Falagas, Zarkadoulla, Ionnidou, Peppas, et al., 2007).

Pinquart and Duberstein based their meta-analysis on 87 studies to investigate the association between perceived social support, network size, marital status, and cancer survival. They found that the reports of individual studies were inconsistent. They reported on a qualitative study that did find that seven studies found a positive association of social involvement and/or social support with the longevity of cancer patients. However, another eight studies failed to find such an association. The subjects had a mean age of 65.9 years, 57% were women, 86% were married, and 14.3% belonged to ethnic minorities.

The fact that the effects of a social network could be biologically mediated was noted by the authors. Social support may limit or mitigate the effects of stress-related endocrine changes possibly associated with tumour proliferation. To cite another example of effective social support, the social network may have a positive influence on health behaviour. An example would be when a married person was prompted to seek an early diagnosis. Social support may also enable one to access the healthcare system more effectively and may facilitate navigating a very complex system. Patients with social support may be more successful in receiving vigorous and active cancer treatment.

The findings of the meta-analysis found support for an association between social support and mortality in cancer patients. Lower mortality in individuals was related to higher levels of perceived social support, a larger social network, and being married. In controlled studies, married respondents had a 12% lower risk than the relative risk for mortality in unmarried persons. The main conclusions reached were that the longevity of cancer patients was related to their perception of social support, the size of their network, and their marital status. The authors concluded: 'The present meta-analysis provides clear and unequivocal evidence for the association of social network with longevity of cancer patients. Reductions of relative risk for mortality by 12–25% in patients with high levels of perceived social support, large social networks and in married persons (controlled studies) show that the effects are clearly clinically meaningful, even though they may be too small to detect in studies that are not sufficiently powered.'

Falagas and associates (2007), in their systematic review of the research literature on the effect of psychosocial factors on the outcome of breast cancer based their findings on 37 studies involving 61,611 female patients. They identified a host of factors, such as role function, fighting spirit, joy, depression, perceived social support, social support, minimization, participation in religious/non-religious groups, and marriage among other factors that were associated with survival/recurrence. It must be noted that these findings emerged mostly from a very few studies specific to each variable. For example, the value of marriage was based on three studies. Their overall conclusion was that the 'parameters associated with better breast cancer prognosis are social support, marriage, minimizing and denial.' They also observed that the actual psychosocial variables associated with survival were inconsistently measured across studies. Both these reviews point to the need for more research predicated on improved methodology.

The power of marriage to prolong life for cancer patients has been noted in both these reviews. In the section that follows, we examine some of the more recent literature on the role of social support to mitigate depression in breast cancer patients. The primacy of social support in moderating depression was reported earlier, in chapter 6. There is some literature that shows that those breast cancer patients who develop depression, among other factors, are lacking in social support (Karakoyun, Gorken, Sahin, Orchin, et al., 2009; Lueboonthavatchai, 2007). In the following section we discuss the role of social support and the social network in the early stages of breast cancer (Burgess, Cornelius, Love, Graham, Richards, & Ramirez, 2005; Gagliardi, Vespa, Papa, Mariotti, Cascinu, & Rossini, 2009), partner support and depression post-mastectomy (Kudel, Edwards, Raja, Haythornthwaite, & Heinberg, 2008), and family support and depression in breast cancer patients (Nausheen & Kamal, 2007).

Gagliardi and associates (2009) conducted a study to investigate the areas of depression, anxiety, and social support using the structural model of the social network. They compared the social network and social support of breast cancer patients with a control group of healthy women. The breast cancer group consisted of 47 women aged between 40 and 65 years with a confirmed diagnosis of breast cancer at low or intermediate-high risk. Most of the patients (80%) were newly diagnosed, and the rest had been ill for between four months and two years. The control group consisted of 58 healthy women and were matched for age, education, marital status, and working situation. Standardized instruments were used to measure social support and social network. Comprehensive demographic information was also collected.

Predictably, anxiety and depression were higher in the breast cancer group compared to the controls. Both groups described strong relationships and had strong ties. However, the breast cancer women described smaller and dense networks, mainly comprising their kin. The healthy women, by contrast, had more friends and co-workers in their network. Surprisingly, no differences emerged between the groups in terms of total support received, which suggested that the presence of a serious medical condition had no impact on the type of support received.

Noteworthy was the finding that differences emerged in the sources of support for the two groups. For the clinical population, information-al support, emotional support, and socialization came from kin. Both groups received instrumental support from kin. The authors concluded that the clinical group rejected sources other their kin for support main-ly because all other sources of support were usually channelled through their kin. Two main conclusions to emerge from the study were:

1 The results demonstrated the importance of emotional and infor-mational support for the mental well-being of the women with breast cancer; and
2 Women in early stages of cancer seemed to be at a disadvantage from their social support and social network relationships. Further-more, the findings seemed to suggest that, overall, the size of the network shrank for the women with breast cancer. One omission (outside the scope of this investigation) in this study was the power of the buffering effect of social support. Nevertheless, changes in the size and structure of the support system are important aspects of social support and were well illustrated by this study. This, in-deed, has important clinical implications.

The next study (Burgess, Cornelius, et al.) explored the risk factors for and prevalence of depression and anxiety in women with breast cancer of recent onset. These women were treated with a lumpecto-my or by a modified radical mastectomy. Data was collected from 222 women with breast cancer who engaged in comprehensive interviews. Data on depression and anxiety was collected at 21, 39, and 60 months for the period between interviews. The DSM-III was used for diagnos-tic purposes. An intimate confiding relationship was defined as cohab-itation with a partner (with or without sexual intimacy).

Ninety-one per cent (202 of 222) of the women completed the first interview. Nine declined the second interview, seven the third, and one the fourth interview. In total, 170 of the 222 (77%) provided com-plete data, either up to five years or to recurrence. The annual preva-lence for the first to fifth years after diagnosis was 48%, 25%, 22%, and 15% respectively.

Risk factors for anxiety and depression, medium term, were past psychological treatment, the absence of an intimate confiding relation-ship, and an experience of serious non-cancer-related difficulties. In the longer term, depression and anxiety were associated with the lack of an intimate confiding relationship, a younger age, severe non-cancer difficulties, and an earlier episode of anxiety, depression, or both after diagnosis.

The prevalence of depression and anxiety in women with early breast cancer is nearly twice that of the general population. Risk factors identified in this study were generally in line with other studies. The quality of social support predicted better health-related quality of life generally in women who were in remission from breast cancer. Again, the authors recommended that psychological interventions for women with breast cancer should take into account the broader social context in which the cancer occurs. One critical element of that social context is the availability of support in general and an intimate confiding relationship in particular. Again, this study did not specifically test the buffering hypothesis of social support, but provided evidence that, among other factors, an intimate confiding relationship has the power to prevent anxiety and depression in early-stage breast cancer patients.

Our next study (Kudel, Edwards, Raja, Haythornthwaite, & Heinberg, 2008) investigated whether marital satisfaction predicted non-weight-related body-image distress, pain impact, and mood in a group of women who had undergone a mastectomy. Five hundred and four women who had undergone a mastectomy at the Johns Hopkins Hospital were mailed a consent form and survey. The response rate was 54% (n=272). The final sample, which included only married women, was 152. The subjects were predominantly white and had some college education. They were 20.85 months post-mastectomy. Among various measures used were the Beck Depression Scale and the Marriage Satisfaction Scale.

The Structural Equation Modeling (SEM) analyses found that higher marital satisfaction was directly or indirectly associated with a positive health outcome. Some of the mechanisms that might have facilitated the outcome were supportive instrumental responses, conversational intimacy, humour, and self-disclosure. Greater marital satisfaction may also decrease the impact of pain when the partner provided direct or instrumental support and helped use more adaptive methods of coping with pain. Similarly, a helpful partner could help the patient adapt to her body image and reduced her fear of disfigurement and the avoidance of intimacy. Another key finding, that the mood of these women improved over time, was a surprise. Possibly mood tended to improve with the passage of time. This was a complex statistical study examining the interrelationships among a host of factors that the authors described as a 'conceptual chain' which increased our understanding of the experiences of women following a mastectomy.

Our final study (Nausheen & Kamal, 2007) was an exploratory study involving 80 Pakistani women with breast cancer. The goal was to study the buffering effect of family social support in protecting the patients against depression. The patients ranged in age from 19 to 74 years (mean age = 42.5 years). All the subjects were married and had children. Forty patients lived in nuclear families, the rest in joint families. No information was provided about their education or income. Seventy-two patients had had a mastectomy.

The Familial Social Support Scale and Siddiqui-Shah Depression Scale were used to obtain data. These scales were available in the Urdu language. The results showed a significant inverse correlation between familial social support and depression. Patients younger than 37 years registered lower scores on depression and higher on familial social support than the older group. Patients with three children or fewer also showed higher familial support. No significant differences emerged for patients living in nuclear and joint families. The main conclusion of this preliminary study was to confirm the buffering hypothesis of social support against depression.

Summary

Spouse/partner support does seem to have a considerable effect in modifying the negative effects of breast cancer. Breast cancer patients, apart from being more vulnerable to depression, experience a whole range of issues related to their body image. This is especially so for those who undergo major surgery such as a radical mastectomy. Being in a stable and long-term relationship appears to be particularly powerful in modifying the negative outcomes associated with breast cancer. The benefits of spousal/partner support ranged from lower mortality, better prognosis, better mental health, lower risk for depression, lower pain levels, and more adaptive coping with cancer. This is a comprehensive list, and research appears to be unanimous in finding support, albeit to varying degrees, for the fact that being married or being in a partner relationship predicts a better outcome for breast cancer patients. This is not to deny that many spouses and partners experience distress in the face of a breast cancer diagnosis and what may follow. Another point of note is the scarcity of literature on the impact of an unsatisfactory marital relationship on coping with breast cancer. Many studies reviewed here also recommended some kind of intervention with the couples going through the experience of breast cancer.

Conclusion

Breast cancer is the most common cancer to afflict women. Over the years the survival rate has steadily risen. This disease has the capacity to create a great deal of distress in the breast cancer sufferer and her intimates. We established that depression is often underestimated in this population. A change in body image, sexuality, deterioration of the quality of life, and young age of the patient contribute to the distress.

Partner-related issues are wide ranging. Yet, there is evidence to the effect that long-term relationships are much less problematic, and indeed a husband or partner is likely to be more supportive. While distress in the partners is relatively common, many partners actually report an improvement in their relationship following the onset of breast cancer. There is some evidence that couples who join support groups report less stress in their relationship. Being married or in a long-term relationship predict a better outcome for breast cancer patients. Husband and partners are often the most powerful source of support for these patients. Many studies recommend some form of intervention with couples.

REFERENCES

American Cancer Society (2007). *Cancer Facts and Figures*. Atlanta: American Cancer Society

Avis, N., Crawford, S., & Manuel, J. (2004). Psychosocial problems among younger women with breast cancer. *Psycho-Oncology, 13*: 295–308.

Baucom, D., Porter, L., Kirby, J., Gremore, T., & Keefe, F. (2006). Psychological issues confronting young women with breast cancer. *Breast Disease, 23*, 103–113.

Brusilovskiy, E., Mitstifer, M., & Salzer, M. (2009). Perceived partner adaptation and psychological outcome for newly diagnosed Stage 1 and Stage II breast cancer patients. *J. Psychosocial Oncology, 27*, 42–58.

Burgess, C., Cornelius, V., Love, S., Graham, J., Richards, M., & Ramirez, A. (2005). Depression and anxiety in women with early breast cancer: Five-year observational cohort study. *BMJ, 330*, 702–705.

Dorval, M., Guay, S., Mondor, M., Masse, B., Falardeau, M., et al. (2005).

Couples who get closer after breast cancer: Frequency and predictors in a prospective investigation. *J. Clinical Oncology., 23,* 3588–3596.

Ellison, L., & Wilkins, K. (2009). Cancer prevalence in the Canadian population. *Statistics Canada: Health Reports, 20,* 7–19.

Falagas, M., Zarkadoulla, E., Ioannidou, E., Peppas, G., Christodoulou, C., & Rafallidis, P. (2007). The effect of psychosocial factors on breast cancer. *Breast Cancer Research, 9,* 44–49.

Feldman, B., & Broussard, A. (2006). Men's adjustment to their partners' breast cancer: A dyadic coping perspective. *Health & Social Work, 31,* 117–127.

Finn, J., Thomas-Rich, A., Katon, W., Cowley, D., et al. (2008). Major depression after breast cancer: A review of epidemiology and treatment. *General Hospital Psychiatry, 30,* 112–126.

Gagliardi, C., Vespa, A., Papa, R., Mariotti, C., Cascinu, S., & Rossini, S. (2009) Social support networks and depression in women suffering from early stage breast cancer: A case control study. *J. Psychosocial Oncology, 27,* 216–229.

Grunfeld, E., Coyle, D., Whelan, T., Clinch, J., et al. (2004). Family caregiver burden: Results of a longitudinal study of breast cancer patients and their principal caregivers. *CMAJ, 170,* 1795–1801.

Henselmans, I., Sanderman, R., Bass, P., Smink, A., & Ranchor, A. (2009). Personal control after a breast cancer diagnosis: Stability and adaptive value. *Psycho-Oncology, 18,* 104–108.

Hodges, L., Humphries, G., & MacFarlane, G. (2005). A meta-analytic investigation of the relationship between the psychological distress of cancer patients and their careers. *Social Science and Medicine, 60,* 1–12.

Hoga, L., Mello, D., & Dias, A. (2008). Psychosocial perspectives of the partners of breast cancer patients treated with a mastectomy. *Cancer Nursing, 31,* 318–325.

Karakoyun, C., Gorken, S., Sahin, S., Orcin, E., Alanyali, H., & Kinay, M. (2009). Depression and anxiety levels in women under follow-up for breast cancer: Relationship to coping with cancer and quality of life. *Medical Oncology* (e-pub., in press).

Kim, Y., Kashy, D., Wellisch, D., Spillers, D., Kaw, C., & Smith, T. (2008). Quality of life of couples dealing with cancer: Dyadic and individual adjustment among breast and prostate cancer survivors and their spousal caregivers. *Annals of Behavior Medicine, 35,* 230–238.

Kudel, I., Edwards, R., Raja, S., Haythornthwaite, J., & Heinberg, L. (2008). The association of perceived support, partner-related social support with self-reported outcomes in women post-mastectomy. *J. Health Psychology, 13,* 1030–1039.

Lueboonthavatchai, P. (2007). Prevalence and psychosocial factors of anxiety and depression in breast cancer patients. *J. Medical Association of Thailand, 90*, 2164–2174.

Manne, S., Ostroff, J., Norton, T., Fox, K., Goldstein, L., & Grana, G. (2006). Cancer-related relationship communication in couples coping with breast cancer. *Psycho-Oncology, 15*, 234–247.

Nausheen, B., & Kamal, A. (2007). Familial social support and depression in breast cancer: An exploratory study on a Pakistani sample. *Psycho-Oncology, 16*, 859–862.

Pinquart, M., & Duberstein, P. (2010). Associations of social networks with cancer mortality: A meta-analysis. *Critical Reviews in Oncology/Hematology, 75*, 122–137.

Shands, M., Lewis, F., Sinsheimer, J., & Cochrane, B. (2006). Core concerns of couples living with breast cancer. *Psycho-Oncology, 15*, 1055–1064.

Skerrett, K. (1998). Couple adjustment to the experience of breast cancer. *Families, Systems & Health, 16*, 281–296.

Wagner, C., Bigatti, S., & Storniolo, A. (2006). Quality of life of husbands of women with breast cancer. *Psycho-Oncology, 15*, 109–120.

Yankaskas, B. (2006). Epidemiology of breast cancer in young women. *Breast Disease, 23*, 3–8.

8 HIV/AIDS and Social Support:
A Troubled Zone

Introduction

HIV/AIDS is by far the most devastating epidemic to emerge in the twentieth century. It is global in scope and is responsible for the deaths of millions of people, mostly in the African continent. At the time of writing, it continues to plague a significant portion of the globe, though in the developed countries this epidemic is under better control and the patients afflicted with HIV/AIDS are living longer. Living with HIV/AIDS is becoming somewhat analogous to living with any chronic condition.

Great progress has been made in dispelling many myths that gave rise to widespread fear about the ease with which the disease was spread. The stigma associated with HIV/AIDS is on the wane, certainly in Western countries, but ignorance and fear continue to persist in many parts of the world (Mahajan, Sayles, Patel, Remien, et al., 2008).

Because of the international scope of HIV/AIDS, the issue of social support assumes extraordinary complexity. The literature is complex and substantial. For that reason, we confine our review to the United States. A rather discouraging conclusion was reached in a recent paper on the epidemiology of HIV/AIDS in the United States and Canada (Hall, Geduld, Boulos, Rhodes, et al., 2009). The rates of HIV transmission in Canada and the United Stated continued to remain high, as overall diagnosis rates have not declined in recent years. Data for this study was derived from HIV/AIDS diagnoses for 1996–2005 reported to the US and Canadian national surveillance systems (33 states in the United States) to determine trends in HIV/AIDS diagnoses and to identify population groups most affected by HIV. The AIDS diagnosis rate was higher in minority groups in both countries (54.1 per 1000 in Blacks and 18.0 in Hispanics compared with 5.9 in Whites in the United States, and 4.7 in Blacks and 4.9 in aboriginal peoples compared with 0.7 in Whites in Canada).

The HIV/AIDS demographics have undergone a dramatic shift over the past twenty years (Centers for Disease Control and Prevention, 2003). HIV/AIDS was predominantly identified among white men engaging in sexual activities with other men. Now heterosexual women are increasingly at risk. The prevalence estimates of HIV/AIDS among women moved from 14% to 22% of adults by the end of 2003. The most significant rise has been in African American and Hispanic women, who accounted for only 25% of all women in the United States, but represented 83% of the AIDS diagnoses in 2003. The rise of new infections in young people between the ages of 13 and 24 is marked and accounts for 12% of individuals diagnosed with HIV/AIDS in 2003 (ibid.).

Psychosocial problems abound in the lives of HIV/AIDS patients. This was demonstrated in a qualitative study based on extensive interviews of HIV/AIDS sufferers (Bogart, Catz, Kelly, Gray-Bernhardt, et al., 2000). Data was obtained from 44 diverse ethnically (43% White, 50% African-American, 5% Hispanic, and 2% Native American) men and living with HIV/AIDS. The mean educational level of the subjects was 13 years. The sample consisted of 37 men and 7 women. The subjects were aware of their HIV status for 70 months on average.

Ten areas explored in this study were: affect, alcohol/drug use, illness experience, life-events, medication, sexual activity, social support, spirituality, and treatment. The illness experience was, at best, mixed. Even among those who reported a positive outcome, such as improved quality of life, many had doubts about their future. These individuals were also depressed. Thoughts of hopelessness were common. Many were also disappointed with their treatment (antiretroviral therapy or HAART) because of the pronounced side-effects. Even taking medication could be an ordeal, as this was a daily reminder of their illness. For many, daily life was structured around taking medication. The authors concluded that individuals who were tired of taking their medication reported a poorer quality of life and wondered if the price of having the side-effects outweighed the benefits of treatment.

Apart from the ill effects of HAART, many patients were despondent about their poor quality of life, especially if they were on disability benefits. Many wished to return to work. Critically, while they enjoyed better health due to their treatment, they were also bored and often had little to occupy their time. Many had financial problems. On the interpersonal front, there were many issues. Most subjects were committed to avoiding sexual relations, especially if they wanted a long-term relationship. Many had disclosed their medical status at the very beginning of a relationship. Many were in emotionally helpful relationships, where the partners helped with keeping medical appointments and reminding them to take medication. Most respondents had concerns about transmitting the disease to their partners and remained celibate, while others used condoms.

Social support presented a mixed picture. A diagnosis of HIV/AIDS elicited both negative and positive responses from friends and relatives. Many patients were helped through their illness by their family members. Nevertheless, there were also numerous examples of discrimination that the subjects experienced at the hands of their friends, family members, and even healthcare professionals. There were examples of family members who made sure that their children were not near the patients. Depression often ensued, as they could no longer trust these people. Fear of discrimination prevented some of the patients from disclosing their condition to family and friends. One way to receive social support was not to disclose their illness.

The authors concluded that this 'research illuminates some of the psychosocial issues and cultural contexts of men and women coping with HIV, particularly issues related to new HIV treatments' (p. 515). Supportive social networks enabled some of the participants to disclose there serostatus to potential partners. Women in this study, however, were more reluctant to disclose and were accepting of celibacy. The authors also noted that a qualitative study could not answer questions related to the prevalence of these issues in the general HIV-positive population.

One key question is, given the levels of prejudice and misinformation about HIV/AIDS, are there barriers to effective social support? Serovich, Brucker, and Kimberly (2000) tested the 'barrier' theory of perceived social support to HIV-positive gay men. The barrier theory proposes that an individual must overcome obstacles to access social support from family. Such barriers might include a lack of acceptance, lack of intimacy, wanting to protect family members, and negative interactions. The authors noted that research revealed that family members were not viewed as helpful for HIV-positive individuals. By contrast, there was substantial evidence showing the supportive role of friends.

This study investigated the uniqueness of social support provided by friends and family members. A total of 134 HIV-positive men were recruited. They were tested for disclosure, relationship satisfaction, social network availability, social support, depression, and physical symptom severity. The hypothesis related to friends in the social network that barriers were predictors of perceived social support was partly supported. The number of friends in the support network was a significant predictor of perceived social support. This indicated that the number of friends to whom the subject had disclosed was also a predictor of more social support. Barriers to social support did not moderate the relationship between perceived social support and depression.

The hypothesis that barriers to disclosure predicted perceived social support from family was supported. One critical finding was that a decrease in the barrier to disclosure predicted perceived social support from family. Perceived social support received from family members was a significant predictor of depression. However, perceived family social support was not a predictor of physical-symptom severity. Levels of satisfaction predicted social support from family, but not friends. Yet, the difference in barriers to family and friends was nominal. The larger the support system available to the HIV-positive men, the less vulnerable they felt. Who the source of support was seemed less important. Discussing the clinical implications of the study, the authors recommended that healthcare professionals involved in HIV/AIDS treatment must identify barriers and develop strategies to remove them.

Family social support is a critical component of anyone's support system. For HIV/AIDS patients this support may not be readily available. This observation was supported in a study of mothers living with HIV/AIDS and their family functioning (Murphy, Marelich, Dello Stritto, Swendeman, & Witkin, 2002). It should be acknowledged that family functioning is a rather under-researched area. This study involved 135 mothers in Los Angeles County with an HIV/AIDS diagnosis or who had symptoms associated with HIV. These mothers had at least one child between the ages of six and eleven. The mothers were assessed for anxiety and depression, health worries and physical functioning, maternal social support, life-events and stressors, and conflict and family functioning. The mean age of the mothers was 34.7 years. The average number of people living in the household was 4.16, of whom 2.38 were children; 73% were living in their own household, 15% with parents or relatives, and 11% in some form of shelter. They were poor, with an average annual income of $14,000.

Mothers were well below the clinical levels of depression. However, even moderate levels of depression had an adverse impact on their relationship with the children and led to poorer family cohesion. Depression also resulted in the mothers not fulfilling family-related tasks. The authors noted that even a modest level of depression could negatively affect family functioning, such as through heightened conflict with the significant other and lower family cohesion. It is noteworthy that disease severity alone did not have significant effect on two dimensions (cohesion and sociability) of family functioning. As for social support, mothers, on average, had three individuals they could count on for physical help, two individuals they could confide in, and no one that interfered with their role as a good mother. In short, the mood state of the mothers emerged as a greater predictor of poor family function than any other factors. The findings of this study are somewhat counter-intuitive, as one might expect these mothers to be more isolated given their medical condition and economic situation.

A number of studies have reported a problematic relationship that HIV/AIDS sufferers and their caregivers' experience with their family members (Smith & Rapkin, 1996; Turner, Pearlin, & Mullan, 1998). Smith and Rapkin identified a number of barriers, which were empirically supported, that interfered with the process of obtaining family support. These included emotional cost, which meant relinquishing ties that were emotionally burdensome. A potential loss of independence, overprotectiveness of family members, and fears of burdening loved ones were also potential barriers. These factors came into play as the disease progressed. The authors summed up the barriers as interpersonal cost, lack of access, lack of acceptance, lack of intimacy, negative interactions, and fear of disclosure. Ciamborne (2002), in a qualitative study of 37 women with HIV/AIDS, found at least one person, usually a family member, on whom they could depend for emotional support. However, with the progression of the disease, the author speculated, informal sources of social support were likely to diminish. A review of the literature on the availability of family-of-origin social support for gay men with AIDS found a striking absence of such support (Kadushin, 1996).

Hall (1999), in a major review of the research literature on the relationship between social support and health in gay HIV-positive men, noted that 'overall, the social support of friends and partners, rather than family of origin, has been found to be more important' (p. 79). This review showed that friends and partners were more likely to respond positively to the disclosure of HIV status than immediate family members. Support from friends and partners also predicted less anxiety and depression. While initially in the disease process family support may be available, it tended to dissipate with the progression of the illness. HIV/AIDS patients also were inclined to seek support from friends and partners to share their concerns about death. However, as death became more imminent, perceived positive family support was more effective in reducing anxiety about death than support from friends.

Finally, Prachakul and Grant (2003), in their review of the literature on informal caregivers of HIV/AIDS patients, found that the majority of caregivers were young adult males, which distinguished them from the characteristics of caregivers of other chronic diseases. The demographic characteristics of caregivers of HIV/AIDS patients were unique. The majority were young Caucasian males who were partners, lovers, or friends and dwelled in large cities, many of whom were seropositive. The authors noted that due to sampling problems, it was difficult to be conclusive about the characteristics of informal caregivers.

Summary

Despite considerable progress in the treatment of HIV/AIDS, the rate of prevalence continues to be high in Canada and the United States. There has been a major shift in the disease's demographics from gay men to minority women and younger persons. Social and psychological problems are endemic to HIV/AIDS sufferers, for whom social support can be both elusive and problematic, and family support suspect. The major source of social support appears to be friends and partners, who are often seropositive. Disclosure to family members remains an issue. HIV/AIDS sufferers encounter numerous barriers to obtaining social support. In the following section, we examine the impact of social support on mitigating depression and other problems associated with depression in HIV/AIDS sufferers.

Social Support for Depression in HIV/AIDS Patients

The literature on HIV/AIDS social support and social network is vast and simply beyond the scope of this chapter. For that reason, the rest of this chapter is devoted to an overview of recent and selected literature on the role of social support for the HIV/AIDS population in the mitigation of depression and problems associated with being depressed.

Ciesla and Roberts (2001), in a meta-analysis of the relationship between HIV infection and the risk for depressive disorders, found strong evidence that HIV infection was associated with an elevated risk for a major depressive disorder. Their meta-analysis, which included ten studies, found a moderate effect size (0.69), which translated into the risk for major depression for HIV-infected patients being 1.99 times higher than for HIV-negative individuals. Contrary to their hypothesis, persons with advanced HIV disease were not different in the rates of major depression than HIV-positive asymptomatic individuals. They concluded that the rate of major depressive disorder in the general HIV-positive population was at the upper end of the 4 to 9% range suggested in previous studies. Rabkin and associates (1997) estimated that lifetime rates of major depression in at-risk HIV cohorts were as high as 50%. Lesserman in a recent article (2008) made the observation that high rates of depression can be accounted for by a growing proportion of HIV population being women and people living in poverty. Both these populations are vulnerable for depressive disorders.

The prevalence of depression and psychiatric illness in the HIV/AIDS population is significant (Benton, 2008; Owe-Larsson, Sall, Salamon, & Allgulander, 2009). Benton found that the prevalence estimates derived from epidemiologic studies of depression in HIV-positive individuals range from a low of 4% to almost 22% for HIV-positive men, and from 2% to 18% for HIV-positive women. Benton (2008) also reported on a recent study that found that in a sample of 2864 HIV-positive patients, almost half were identified as having some form of psychiatric illness, more than one-third of the sample were positive for major depression, and more than one-quarter were positive for dysthymia. Depression can have many and varied consequences on the lives of HIV/AIDS patients.

In a well-designed study, Simoni, Huang, Goodry, and Montoya (2005) reported on the benefits of social support in a group of 373 mainly African American and Puerto Rican HIV-positive women. Of the subjects, 44% African American, 42% Hispanic, and 11% of mixed ethnicity. On average they had 11 years of schooling and the average family income was $1000 per month. This was a disadvantaged group. Just over 53% were currently in a relationship. The rest were single or never legally married. These women were assessed for depression, social support, self-esteem, and mastery.

A full 61% were above the cut-off point for depression on the Center for Epidemiological Studies for Depression (CES-D) scale. The prediction that frequency of receiving HIV-related social support (information and advice, tangible assistance, encouragement and reassurance, and listening and attempting to understand) would be negatively related to depression was supported. The relationship between social support and depressive symptomatology was mediated by what was described as psychological resourcefulness, which comprised self-esteem and mastery. Persons in receipt of social support experienced an increase in self-esteem and decrease in psychological distress. The model in this study showed that the variance in depressive symptomatology mediated by psychological resourcefulness was 55.8%. The authors emphasized the need to assess HIV-positive women for social isolation and depression and to provide them with interventions such as support groups that would capitalize on their existing strengths, including their psychological resourcefulness.

McDowell and Serovich (2007) reported a complex study that explored the differential impact on their mental health of perceived and real social support in three groups, gay men, straight or bisexual men, and women living with HIV/AIDS. The participants in this study were 125 women and 232 men with an HIV-positive or AIDS diagnosis. They completed questionnaires regarding mental health, social support, physical health, disease progression, and sexual risk-taking behaviours once every six months over three years, resulting in seven data collection points.

Women in this study were mostly African American (68%), with a mean age of 37.74 years. Gay men were mostly white (68%) with a mean age of 37.70 years, and straight and bisexual men were primarily African American with a mean age of 40.7 years. In terms of education, employment, and income there were major differences between the groups. For instance, 47% of the gay men had college and graduate degrees compared to 8% of the women. Similar differences were also evident in income. A full 38% of gay men had income ranging between $1501 and $2000 or more per month. For women this figure was 15.2%; 66.4% refused to answer this question.

In terms of social support, gay men reported less actual support from family than did women and straight and bisexual men. However, no significant difference was noted between the three groups in relation to social support from friends. Significant differences emerged between the three groups on perceived social support from family and friends. Education had a significant association with friends and race was significantly associated with social support from family.

For HIV-positive women, perceived social support from family was critical. The authors speculated that women may be more socialized than men to expect support from family members. Most critically, significant differences emerged in the relationship between perceived and actual social support and mental health. Perceived social support had the most predictive power of mental health indices, but depressive symptoms and loneliness over the past few days in gay men were predicted by actual support from family. Authors postulated that although gay men seemingly had more friends in their support system, access to family members seemed to influence the depression and loneliness experienced by them. This last finding provides indirect support for the proposition that the desire for family support seems to increase as male HIV/AIDS patients approach death (Hall, 1999).

McDowell and Serovich (2007) conducted an important study that focused on the relationship between mental health and social support in three groups who were demographically very divergent. It adds significantly to our understanding of the complexities that surround the subject of social support. The sample sizes were large, and overall, despite some limitations in measurements, the study was methodologically well designed.

In the following two studies we examine, among other factors, the interactional effects of social support, depression, and adherence to medical treatment for HIV/AIDS patients (Gonzalez, Penedo, Antoni, Duran, et. al., 2004; Vyavaharkar, Moneyham, Tavakoli, Phillips, et al., 2007).

Gonzalez and associates investigated HIV treatment adherence in men and women living with HIV/AIDS. Their groundbreaking study examined the complexity of the relationships between social support, psychological state, and HIV-treatment. Subjects were drawn from the population of HIV/AID patients involved in a larger study at the University of Miami. The participants were 90 HIV-positive men who had sex with men and women of any sexual orientation. The subjects were between the ages of 18 and 65 years. They used the following measurement instruments: a questionnaire on demographics and health-related variables; a Social Provision Scale that had six constructs of social-relationship provision (attachment, social integration, opportunity for nurturance, reassurance of worth, reliable alliance, and guidance); Beck Depression Inventory (BDI), a 21-item questionnaire that measures the severity of depressive symptoms; the Psychological State of Mind scale (PSOM), which measures persons' capacities to enter positive cognitive and interpersonal states over the past week; and the Adherence to Combination Therapy Guide, which measures medication adherence and immune measures.

The mean age of the subjects was 39.4 years and the mean duration of HIV diagnosis was 67.6 months. The subjects were on antiretrovirals for 1.9 years. Education levels ranged from grades 7–12 to graduate school, and income ranged from under $10,000 to over $50,000 per year. However, 77% of the subjects earned from under $10,000 to $30,000 per annum. As for employment, 41% were employed part-time or full-time, 32% were disabled, and another 19% were unemployed.

Several findings were in the predictable direction. The social support measure used in this study did not specify the persons and their relationship with the subjects or frequency of contact. Perceived quality of social support was significantly related to medication adherence even after controlling for alcohol consumption and age. Perceived quality of social support was also associated with lower depressive symptoms and higher levels of PSOM. PSOM and depression were individually related to medication adherence. The higher the levels of depressive symptomatology, the lower was the adherence to medication. Predictably, the higher the levels of PSOM, the higher were the levels of medication adherence. One novel finding of this study was the finding that PSOM was a significant predictor of medication adherence. The authors noted that this was a new construct and deserved further replication.

Vyavaharkar and associates (2007) also investigated the relationship between social support and medication adherence. This study had several unique features. It involved only HIV-positive women who were clinically depressed and living in rural areas of the south-eastern United States. The sample consisted of 224 women who were all HIV-positive and residing in ten rural communities. They had to score 16 points (cut-off point for depression) or higher on the CES-D scale.

Instrument used in this study were as follows: the Medical Outcomes Study Social Support Survey, which measured chronically ill subjects' perception of the availability of social support and the Social Support Questionnaire (SSQ6), which measured the sources of support and satisfaction with social support; and the Family Coping Project Coping Scale (FCPCS), which measured coping responses. Medication adherence was measured by two proxy variables (self-reported missed HIV medications and reasons for missed medications in the past month). Of the 224 women in this study, 133 (59.38%) were non-compliant with their drug regimens at least once during the preceding month. Medication adherence has been recognized as a particular problem among rural HIV-positive women.

Two variables, coping by denial and the number of children, were positively correlated with reasons for missed medication, while availability of social support, coping by spiritual activities, managing HIV disease, positive thinking, focusing on others, and focusing on the present were negatively correlated with reasons for missed medication. Social support and coping emerged as particularly powerful predictors of medical adherence. However, social support lost some power when coping variables were added to the models, with the coping variables emerging as significant predictors of adherence. As for the effectiveness of social support, the authors reported that the findings did not provide any insight into the actual types of support that may promote medication adherence in the HIV population. They further observed that it was not the mere availability of social support, but the satisfaction with the available social support which was more effective for medication adherence. Overall, satisfaction with available social support combined with coping by managing HIV disease were the best positive predictors of medication adherence. The intricate nature of the relationship between medication adherence, depression, and HIV/AIDS was evident in a study by Gibbie, Hay, Hutchinson, and Mijch (2007). They found that while depression was not directly associated with adherence, being in a relationship increased the likelihood of non-adherence, while living with other people predicted adherence to HAART. Social support emerged as a significant predictor of medication adherence in all the above studies. However, there were major differences as to the source of that support.

The final two reports involve the role of social and emotional support in minority women living with HIV/AIDS in New York City (Simoni & Cooperman, 2000) and men living with HIV (Deichert, Fekete, Boarts, Druley, & Delahanty, 2008). Simoni and Cooperman conducted a project involving 373 women living with HIV/AIDS in New York City. The primary objective of this study was to study and understand women's psychological adaptation to living with HIV/AIDS. This was a non-probability sample, and the subjects, who were primarily African American or Latino, were interviewed face-to-face by the investigators. Their mean age was 39.61 years. The majority of the women were either never married (52%), legally married (12%), separated (14%), divorced (11%), or widowed (11%). Most women

(74%) were heterosexual. Most were poor (85% reporting less than $1000 per month income).

The following measures were used. Frequencies of physical and sexual abuse below the age of 16 and since then were used to measure trauma. A checklist was used to assess substance abuse. Stressors (trauma) were assessed using the frequencies of sexual and physical abuse below the age of 16 and since that age. Strength was measured by a 13-item scale of Somali on spirituality. Social support was measured by a modified version of the UCLA Social Support Inventory; this scale was used to assess HIV-related support.

The results revealed high levels of both stressors and strengths in these women. A full 59% and another 69% were sexually and physically abused respectively. The mean score on CES-D was 21.36, and a full 61% scored over 16, the cut-off point for depression. As for their physical state, 34% had minimal symptoms and 41% were asymptomatic. Health over the previous 30 days was considered poor by 13%, fair by 31%, good by 26%, and very good by 18%. Strengths (spirituality, mastery) showed an association with both psychological and physical adaptation. The beneficial effects of spirituality on depression seemed to be mediated by mastery. Social support proved to be a major factor in showing better psychological and physical health. The authors postulated that, on the basis of their analysis, social support may indeed buffer gay women from the pernicious effects of earlier trauma. Some of the limitations of this study were that the population was a sample of convenience and that all the data were self-reported, which usually poses questions about its reliability. Despite the methodological shortcomings, we chose to include this study because of the very vulnerable population investigated, who were also confronted with almost insurmountable odds. This study, minimally, was able to show the power of social support and personal strength to mitigate some of the struggles of living with HIV/AIDS.

Our final study (Deichert, Fekete, Boarts, Druley, & Delahanty, 2008) was a cross-sectional investigation of the complex relationship between affect, social support, and adjusting to living with HIV/AIDS. The participants were 105 men over the age of 18 who were either HIV-positive or diagnosed with AIDS, and who had a primary provider of support. The mean age of the subjects was 39.2 years. Most were African American (48.6%), followed by Caucasian (37.1%), Hispanic (12.2%), Asian (1.0%) and Indian (1.0%). Most were unemployed (61.6%) and reported an average monthly income of $1000. Most of the men were gay (60%).

The following measures were used: Emotional Support Scale, CES-D, Positive and Negative Affect Schedule, General Health Behaviors Measure, and Ways of Coping Scale.

The findings were complex. Higher levels of emotional support were related to engaging in more health behaviours. Emotional support also accounted for less depression, and higher positive affect resulted in more active coping. Further analysis revealed that the link between emotional support and health behaviours failed to reach a statistically significant result after accounting for the effects of depression. Depression and positive affect may very well be separate pathways through which support functions on men's ability to cope with their illness. The authors concluded that emotional support was associated with engaging in greater levels of health behaviours and active coping efforts in men living with HIV. Depression and positive affect were separate pathways through which support operated on men's ability to manage their illness. Positive affect seemed to enhance men's ability to cope more effectively with the stressors associated with HIV/AIDS, and fewer symptoms of depression seemed to lead to engaging in healthy behaviours. This study once again attested to the complexity of relationships among multiple factors that begin to explain the complicated nature of the relationships between the critical factors that affect the lives of HIV/AID patients.

Summary

Depressive disorder and depressive symptoms are relatively common in the HIV/AIDS population. The estimates of prevalence of depressive disorder vary from a low of 4% to a high of 33% (Benton, 2008). There is general consensus in the literature that the HIV/AIDS population is vulnerable for depression for both biological and psychosocial reasons.

Depression in HIV/AIDS sufferers further complicates their clinical picture. While pharmacological treatment is often effective for depression, social factors such as social support also play a significant role in its amelioration. The relationship between depression and HIV/AIDS is complex and is influenced by a multitude of factors. Still, the selected studies that we discussed point to the positive power of social support. Factors such as psychological resourcefulness, demographic factors, and the availability of support all exert an influence on the effectiveness of social support to mitigate depression in this population.

There also exist interesting differences between gay men and women in their sources of social support. Gay men receive much of their support from friends and partners, who are often seropositive. Women, by contrast, rely more on family members. Finally, what is truly noteworthy is how the efficacy of social support is ultimately determined by a whole host of factors that interact with each other in a very complex way. Social support also has a major influence on medication adherence in HIV/AIDS sufferers, who may also be depressed.

Conclusion

HIV/AIDS continues to be a major public health issue. In the United States and Canada, the prevalence of HIV/AIDS continue to rise. The population affected by this infection has shifted away from gay men to African American and Hispanic women. The social problems encountered by this HIV/AIDS population are multi-dimensional and complex. Poverty in this population remains high. Depression is also endemic to the HIV/AIDS population.

Social support presents a different face in relation to HIV/AIDS than to almost any other chronic illness. Family as a source of social support remains elusive for gay men with HIV/AIDS. Friends and partners often seropositive themselves are the main sources of social support for these men. The picture is somewhat different for women. They are more likely to have family support. Depression in this population further complicates the social support question. The availability of social support alone may not in itself mitigate depression or lead to better coping. There is, however, some evidence that social support promotes medication adherence. Satisfaction with the available support seems to be a determining factor in terms of its effectiveness. Personal strengths, specific types of support such as emotional support, spirituality, support from family members vis-à-vis friends or male partners, and other factors influence the effectiveness of social support. However, our review confirmed the power of social support in coping with the problems of living with HIV/AIDS.

REFERENCES

Benton, T. (2008). Depression and HIV/AIDS. *Current Psychiatric Reports, 10*, 280–285.
Bogart, L., Catz, S., Kelly, J., Gray-Bernhardt, M., et al. (2000). Psychosocial

issues in the era of new AIDS treatment from the perspective of persons living with HIV. *J. Health Psychology, 5*, 500–516.

Centers for Disease Control and Prevention (2003). HIV/AIDS Surveillance
Report, 15: 1–46. http://www.cdc.gov/hiv/surveillance/resources/
reports/2003report/.

Ciambrone, D. (2002). Informal networks among women with HIV/AIDS:
Present support and future prospects. *Qualitative Health Research, 12*,
876–896.

Ciesla, J., & Roberts, J. (2001). Meta-analysis of the relationship between HIV
infection and risk for depressive disorders. *Am. J. Psychiatry, 158*, 725–730.

Deichert, N., Fekete, E., Boarts, J., Druley, J., & Delahanty, D. (2008). Emotional
support and Affect: Associations with health behaviors and active coping
efforts in men living with HIV/AIDS. *Behavior, 12*, 139–145.

Gibbie, T., Hay, M., Hutchinson, C., & Mijch, A. (2007). Depression, social support and adherence to highly active antiretroviral therapy in people living
with HIV/AIDS. *Sexual Health, 4*, 227–232.

Gonzalez, J., Penedo, F., Antoni, M., Duran, R., et al. (2004). Social support,
positive states of mind, and HIV treatment adherence in men and women
living with HIV/AIDS. *Health Psychology, 23*, 413–418.

Hall, H., Geduld, J., Boulos, D., Rhodes, P., et al. (2009). Epidemiology of HIV
in the United States and Canada: Current status and ongoing challenges. *J.
Acquired Immune Deficiency Syndromes, 51*, S13–S20.

Hall, V. (1999). The relationship between social support and health in gay men
with HIV/AIDS: An integrative review. *J. Association of Nurses in AIDS Care,
10*, 74–8.

Kadushin, G. (1996). Gay men with AIDS and their families of origin: An
analysis of social support. *Health and Social Work, 21*: 141–150.

Lesserman, J. (2008). Role of depression, stress, and trauma in HIV disease
progression. *Psychosomatic Medicine, 70*, 539–545.

Mahajan, A., Sayles, J., Patel, V., Remien, R., et al. (2008). Stigma in the HIV/
AIDS epidemic: A review of the literature and recommendations for the
way forward. *AIDS, 22 (Suppl 2)*, S67–S79.

McDowell, T., & Serovich, M. (2007). The effect of perceived and actual social
support on the mental health of HIV-positive persons. *AIDS Care, 19*,
1223–1229.

Murphy, D., Marelich, W., Dello Stritto, M., Swendeman, D., & Witkin, A.
(2002). Mothers living with HIV/AIDS: Mental, physical, and family functioning. *Aids Care, 14*, 633–644.

Owe-Larsson, B., Sall, L., Salamon, E., & Allgulander,·C. (2009). HIV infection
and psychiatric illness. *African J. Psychiatry, 12*, 115–128.

Prachakul, W., & Grant, J. (2003). Informal caregivers of persons with HIV/
    AIDS: A review and analysis. *J. Association of Nurses in AIDS Care, 14,* 55–71.
Rabkin, J., Ferrando, S., Jacobsberg, L., & Fishman, B. (1997). Prevalence of
    Axis 1 disorders in the AIDs cohort: A cross-sectional controlled study. *Comprehensive Psychiatry, 38,* 146–154.
Serovich, J., Brucker, P., & Kimberly, J. (2000). Barriers to social support for
    persons living with HIV/AIDS. *Aids Care, 12,* 651–662.
Simoni, J., & Cooperman, N. (2000). Stressors, and strengths among women
    with HIV/AIDs in New York City. *AIDS Care, 12,* 291–297.
Simoni, J., Huang, B., Goodry, E., & Montoya, H. (2005). Social support and
    depressive symptomatology among HIV-positive women: The mediating
    role of self-esteem and mastery. *Women and Health, 42,* 1–15.
Smith, M., & Rapkin, B. (1996). Social support and barriers to family involvement in caregiving for persons with AIDS: Implications for patient education. *Patient Education and Counseling, 27,* 85–94.
Turner, H., Pearlin, L., & Mullan, J. (1998). Sources and determinants of social
    support for caregivers of persons with AIDS. *J. Health and Social Behavior, 39,*
    137–151.
Vyavaharkar, M., Moneyham, L., Tavakoli, A., Phillips, K., et al. (2007). Social
    support, coping, and medication adherence among HIV-positive women
    with depression living in rural areas of the south-eastern United States.
    AIDS Patient Care and STDs, 21, 667–680.

9 Social Support and Network Interventions

Introduction

In this chapter we propose to report, first, on social support interventions in general, and second, on interventions with two conditions (breast cancer and dementia) that we discussed in earlier chapters. It must be stated that the literature on social support intervention is huge and we are able to present only a selected sample. Our goal, however, is to make some assessment about the effectiveness of different forms of social support. The range of problems for which social support interventions have been used is astounding: from church-based support to reduce mortality (Krause, 2006) to intervention for the cessation of smoking (May, West, Hajek, McEwen, & McRobbie, 2006) to infant feeding practices (Watt, Tull, Hardy, Wiggins, et al., 2008). We begin by presenting a brief summary of the above studies and some more.

May and colleagues (2006) conducted a large-scale randomized controlled trial to assess the effectiveness of incorporating a buddy system in a group therapy intervention program to promote smoking cessation. Five hundred and sixty smokers were randomly assigned to a group therapy program where each smoker was assigned a friend (buddy) to provide mutual support and the other group's members were without such a buddy. Treatment followed the widely used 'withdrawal-oriented model' of smoking cessation, which has been in use in the United Kingdom for some time.

The results were somewhat equivocal. The effect of the 'buddy' system was in the right direction for about a week after the cessation of smoking, but then over time the effect disappeared. The authors suggested that the level of social support inherent in a group therapy program might have diminished the effects of the pairing with a fellow-smoker. Nevertheless, the effect on abstinence rates of the buddy intervention did increase the individual perception of social support, with the buddy group reporting a greater sense of support and someone to turn to on their date of quitting. However, the longevity of this effect remained unknown.

Some years earlier, May and West (2000) conducted a literature review on the effectiveness of social support interventions (buddy systems) in the cessation of smoking. They encountered serious problems in their selection of studies for inclusion in this review, mainly due to methodological shortcomings. Ten studies were reviewed, but no significant support for the benefits of the 'buddy system' was found. Poorly designed studies accounted for much of the problem with this review. The authors were sanguine that better-designed investigations might very well show the beneficial aspects of a buddy system in the cessation of smoking.

Krause (2006) is not, strictly speaking, a report on social support intervention. Rather, it was an investigation to determine if support provided and received from fellow church members reduced the negative effects of financial strain on mortality. Because of the involvement of an institution such as a church and its acknowledged supportive role for its congregations, we decided to report this study. It was based on a national sample of 1500 older adults in 2001 and 2004. They were asked about their financial situation, church-based social support, and private and public religious practices. In 2004, mortality status was determined in follow-up interviews. The average age of the participants was 74.2 years. In all, 46% were white and 54% were black.

Church attendance was associated with lower mortality. Older individuals, individuals with less education, and those with less-favourable health at the baseline were more likely to die during the follow-up period. Other findings were that attending Bible study classes, prayer groups, and so on resulted in a higher rate of mortality for older adults. As for any interaction between financial stress and church attendance, the results showed that as the level of support increased, the impact of financial strain on mortality decreased. Interestingly, the impact of financial strain on mortality was reduced for older people, who in turn provided more emotional support to the people in their church. In other words, not just receiving social support but providing it also had a positive outcome. Krause warned that the results, while thought-provoking, needed a great deal more research, since only one source of stress, financial strain, was investigated. It would of considerable value to see whether the protective function of providing support to others extended to other kind of stressors.

Watt and associates (2008) conducted a study to assess if monthly home visits by trained volunteers had any beneficial effect on infant feeding practices at age 12 months. To this end, they carried out a randomized, controlled trial with a disadvantaged group in the inner-city London boroughs. Three hundred and twelve babies attending baby clinics were randomized to receive monthly home visits from trained volunteers over a nine-month period. Several nutrition-related outcome measures were established. Data collection occurred at baseline with infants aged about 10 weeks, and in follow-ups at age 12 and 18 months. In all, 212 women completed the trial. No significant differences emerged between the two groups on the principal outcome measure of vitamin C intake. However, at follow-up, infants in the experimental group were less likely to be fed goat's or soya milk. They were also more likely to have three solid meals a day. The authors noted that the strength of this study was its randomized design and the successful implementation of the support intervention by volunteers. They recommended that future work was needed to determine how an effective social intervention program could be incorporated within a broader strategy to address the determinants of infant feeding.

We end this section with two systematic reviews on the benefits of social support intervention on diabetes (van Dam, van der Horst, Knoops, Ryckman, et al., 2005) and mental health problems (Pistrang, Barker, & Humphreys, 2008). Van Dam and associates begin their review by providing useful categories of social support, which include emotional support (warmth and nurturance), appraisal support (helping an individual understand stressful events and what resources are needed to deal with the contingency), informational support (giving appropriate advice and information), and tangible assistance (material or other practical help). After a comprehensive search they found only six controlled studies that met the criteria for inclusion. Their research question was, do methodologically sound studies provide evidence of social support interventions on self-care and health outcomes in type 2 diabetes?

The six studies covered a wide range of interventions such as support from fellow patients versus individual visits, counselling from a nutritionist, group sessions, telephone calls from a peer counsellor versus educational pamphlets received by mail, patients provided with computers and Internet access to diabetes information, Internet-based social support versus Internet access without social support, and monthly group sessions and a diabetes education program versus diabetes education but no group sessions.

The authors noted, first, the rather small number of what may be considered methodologically acceptable studies and, second, that all the studies provided some evidence to support their therapeutic usefulness. The studies were heterogeneous and not comparable. The authors cautioned against drawing any general conclusions. Interventions were also varied. Some general conclusions were possible. Biomedical outcomes were assessed in four studies, two of them providing evidence of positive outcome. Their final conclusion was that the review could not clarify what elements of social support and which mechanisms underlying them were most effective in self-management of type 2 diabetes.

Pistrang and colleagues (2008) conducted a review of psychosocial interventions for the mentally ill based on 12 papers. The target populations in these studies were patients with chronic mental illness, depression/anxiety, and those experiencing bereavement. Only four of the studies included were randomized controlled trials, three were non-randomized trials, four were prospective longitudinal, and three cross-sectional. Five of the 12 studies did not find any significant differences in mental health outcomes between mutual-help group members and non members. Seven studies reported positive changes for those involved in social support groups.

This review, unlike the preceding, is limited by the somewhat loose inclusion criteria (inclusion of non-randomized studies), which made the findings less powerful. Nevertheless, they provided limited and, what the authors describe as, promising evidence of the benefits of mutual self-help groups to bring about positive changes in individuals with mental illness. Two randomized studies in this review showed that mutual help groups were equivalent to more expensive, professionally run group therapy programs.

Summary

The beneficial effects of social support interventions with varied problems and populations was found to be somewhat equivocal. Yet, there was some evidence for optimism. While the 'buddy' system in itself did not significantly lead to smoking cessation, the results were in the right direction. The role of the church in reducing mortality in persons who were financially strained, while promising, did not produce the outcome that was predicted. However, one finding worthy of further investigation was that people who were in the role of helpers experienced prolongation of their lives. Social support interventions with diabetic patients also yielded an encouraging but not significant outcome. One key problem was the small number of rather diverse studies. Mentally ill patients can and do benefit from social support interventions. The problem was that the review of the programs had inherent weaknesses as it included methodologically wanting studies. Our foray into a variety of social support interventions with wide-ranging problems leads us to conclude that much more research is called for before any firm claim about their success or failure can be made.

Breast Cancer and Social Support Interventions

The benefits of social support interventions with breast cancer (among others) patients was brought into question by two recent systematic reviews on that topic (Edwards, Hulbert-Williams, & Neal, 2008; Nausheen, Gidron, Peveler, & Moss-Morris, 2009).

Edwards and colleagues, in a systematic review on the benefits of psychological therapy for women with metastatic breast cancer, concluded that psychological therapies that included cognitive behavioural therapy, educational programs, and group support were of limited value either for psychological support or survival outcomes. This review was based on three support-expressive group therapies and five studies of group psychological therapies. Group therapy programs were led by either patients or professionals. Our interest is in the former.

The supportive/expressive group therapy programs had the objectives of building bonds, expressing emotions, detoxifying death and dying, redefining life-priorities, increasing the support of friends and families, improving the doctor–patient relationship, and improving coping skills. These groups yielded inconsistent outcomes. While the intervention groups did show improved mood, better coping skills, and better pain control, over time these benefits did not last. Survival for the intervention group was significantly higher in the short run. Median survival, however, was unchanged. The authors concluded that there was insufficient evidence to advocate psychological therapies (cognitive behavioural and supportive-expressive) should be made available to women diagnosed with metastatic breast cancer. The benefits appeared to be of a short-term nature.

Nausheen, Gidron, Peveler, and Moss-Morris (2009) in their systematic review of 26 papers on social support and progression of cancer also concluded that while breast cancer yielded the best outcome in terms of a relationship between social support and cancer progression, which was confirmed by five studies, there was insufficient evidence of the value of social support for other types of cancer. Social support in this review was placed into two categories: structural support, which included the quantitative elements of social network such as size, range, bondedness, and proximity; and functional support, which referred to the quality and function of the structural support components such as the provision of informational, emotional, and instrumental support.

The authors noted the importance, to enhance the benefits of therapeutic interventions, of identifying patients who were at risk due to their psychological vulnerabilities resulting from low support. Future research should explore the relevance of improving social support skills to elicit support from the social network to assess its impact on the progression of the disease.

Our next two studies report from two rather different perspectives on the benefits of social support interventions. Napoles-Springer and colleagues (2009) report on an exploratory investigation to determine the need to develop a culturally relevant peer support group for Spanish-speaking Latinos with breast cancer (Napoles-Springer, Ortiz, O'Brien, & Diaz-Mendez, 2009). The other study was a quasi-experimental study to examine the effectiveness of a telephone support system for patients with breast cancer (Salonen, Tarkka, Kellokumpu-Lehtinen, Astedt-Kurki, Luukkaala, et al., 2009).

Napoles-Springer and associates wanted to assess the needs for and barriers to acceptability and effectiveness of psychosocial support services for Latino women with breast cancer. To that end, they explored the benefits of a peer-support counsellor intervention. The analysis was based on 89 women referred for psychosocial services, 29 speaking survivors of breast cancer, and 17 culturally component advocates for the women with breast cancer. The results showed that the Latino women with breast cancer confronted unique sociocultural factors that had to be taken into account for any effective social support intervention. One such problem was simply navigating the complex medical world and language barriers. This often resulted in low-quality information. Peer-support intervention ameliorated many of these problems. The greatest benefits seem to be in the domain of emotional support, and the identity of the peer counsellor as a cancer survivor was of utmost significance.

The authors concluded that emotional and informational support were equally important for their patient population. Early contact following a diagnosis of breast cancer was also found to be of major importance. Initial contact was best made in person to develop trust in the peer counsellor and help reduce anxiety. These women were a disadvantaged group from virtually every point of view and experienced extraordinary levels of hardship. The peer counsellor program for them was invaluable.

Salonen and colleagues (2009) conducted a study to explore the benefits of telephone support intervention a week after surgery for the quality of life of patients with breast cancer. The sample consisted of 228 patients with breast cancer allocated to a treatment group (n=220) and a control (n=120). The patients were quasi-randomized. A number of valid instruments were used to measure quality of life. The intervention group received support from a physiotherapist, with a single telephone call a week after surgery, before any adjuvant treatment began. The phone calls could last from 3 minutes to 25 minutes. The goals of the phone calls were teaching and providing information about the illness, teaching home exercises, giving advice and information, general health education, and developing the therapist–patient relationship, among others.

Almost all the women in the intervention group wanted the telephone support system to continue. However, as far as quality of life was concerned, no significant differences emerged between the treatment and the control groups. The authors also reported on some interesting differences in the women's responses, based on age, to the positive effect of telephone intervention. Older patients seemingly derived more benefits. While statistically the phone intervention did not prove to be any more effective than standard treatment, the authors noted that the clinical benefits could not be ignored. Having the opportunity to ask questions about troubling matters was reported as most helpful.

Summary

The two systematic reviews, while addressing different issues, raised critical questions about the effectiveness of social support interventions. One major issue is the question of outcome in these studies. Very few studies in these reviews shared the same or even similar outcomes. For the authors of these reviews the task of finding studies that could be grouped together was a major challenge. Despite numerous methodological issues, both reviews gave hope about the benefits that could accrue from social support interventions. Our last two studies also testify to that. These two again revealed the sheer scope of social support interventions. Patients do benefit from social support interventions. Improved research methods are needed to further clarify the questions of who are aided and why.

Social Support Interventions for Patients with Dementia and Their Caregivers

Here we examine the effectiveness of social support interventions with patients with dementia and their caregivers. We rely almost entirely on the results of systematic reviews to make a judgment about the effectiveness of social support interventions.

Two very recent systematic reviews have reported on the effectiveness of psychosocial interventions with dementia patients (O'Connor, Ames, Gardner, & King, 2009; Spijker, Vernooij-Dassen, Vasse, Adang, et al., 2008). Spijker and associates conducted a meta-analysis of the literature to determine the effectiveness of social support interventions that would delay the institutionalization of patients with dementia. This was one of the very first systematic reviews on this topic. Altogether 13 studies met the criteria for inclusion. These 13 studies included 9043 patients. Overall, the effectiveness of these programs had significantly reduced the odds of institutionalization, and had significantly increased the time to institutionalization by minimizing healthcare risks. Although all the patients in these studies were community-dwelling, four of these studies were conducted in outpatient settings. Two studies reported treating their patients in their own homes.

Effective interventions had the essential qualities of being multicomponent, 'with a range of specific, supportive caregiving interventions ... Most interventions were individualized, intensive, individualized interventions designed to meet the unique needs of patients and their caregivers' (Spijker et al., p. 1126). Support intervention was provided by counsellors or case mangers who also received specific training. This is an important point, as social support programs are often associated with peer and community support programs. This review reported studies where professionals designed specific programs to promote social support. Interventions offered multiple choices that included counselling and other support services. The authors attributed the success of these programs to the ability of the patients and their caregivers to choose the ones that would lead to their satisfactory involvement. For the support programs to be effective in delaying institutionalization, they had to be intense, with the caregiver and the patient with dementia actively involved in seeking solutions.

The next review, conducted by O'Connor and colleagues (2009), unlike the previous review, had less well-defined outcomes. A variety of psychosocial interventions were involved, which resulted in reducing psychological symptoms in dementia patients, including anxiety, depression, and social withdrawal. Out of some 48 papers, only 12 met the criteria of this review. Both randomized controlled trials (RCTs) and pre-test versus post-test repeated-measure studies were included. Eight of the studies were RCTs. Interventions included music, person-centred care, physical activity, recreation, relaxation, reminiscence therapy, and more.

The results were not encouraging. Some interventions, such as care education, recreation, and validation therapy, were more successful in reducing psychological symptoms than attention control conditions. However, the level of evidence was less than compelling. Many of the improvements could not be categorically attributed to any single treatment condition. The authors concluded that psychological symptoms were difficult to treat irrespective of approach. It is noteworthy that this review was not strictly confined to social support interventions. Some of the interventions included here had elements of social support, while others were more categorically designed to treat psychological symptoms. Our reason for including this review is two-fold: first, systematic reviews of social support interventions with dementia patients are somewhat rare for the simple reason that by definition interventions such as peer-group or network interventions could not effectively be implemented with this population; and second, as stated, some of the interventions, such as music therapy, reminiscence therapy, and person-centred care, may incorporate some elements of social support interventions.

These two systematic reviews also reveal the breadth of outcome associated with psychological and social interventions. Strictly social-support interventions, for patients with dementia – that is, interventions that by definition involve an engagement that explicitly attempts to enhance a patient's source of social support and thereby generate psychosocial benefits – are hard to find. Are social support interventions with the caregivers of patients with dementia any more effective? Presently, we report on three recent systematic reviews on that topic

(Peacock & Forbes, 2003; Powell, Chiu, & Eysenbach, 2008; Thompson, Spilsbury, Hall, Birks, et al., 2007); an RCT on the typology of social support and its relationship to the institutionalization of the person with dementia (Charlesworth, Tzimoula, Higgs, & Poland, 2007); and another RCT that evaluated the effectiveness of a befriending scheme to improve mental health and quality of life for the family caregivers of patients with dementia (Charlesworth, Shepstone, Wilson, Reynolds, et al., 2008).

One of the earlier systematic reviews on the effectiveness of psychosocial interventions, reported by Peacock and Forbes (2003), found a rather discouraging outcome. In all, they identified 36 relevant studies, of which only 11 were methodologically acceptable. A range of interventions were reported by the authors, some of which were strictly psychotherapeutic and educational, administered by professionals, and did not fall into the category of social-support-type interventions. One intervention, however, was a computer-networking intervention that involved receiving information, decision-making support, communication, and an opportunity for questions and answers. The group involved in computer networking demonstrated a significant increase in decision-making confidence. No significant differences, however, emerged between the groups on decision-making skills, social isolation, or the use of health services. The most common outcome measures, reported by the educational and psychotherapeutic interventions, were related to institutionalization of the patient with dementia, followed by death of the patient, behaviour disturbance, caregiver depression, caregiver strain, caregiver stress, and use of formal services.

A major conclusion reached by this review was the limitation of psychological interventions; another was that education-oriented interventions revealed very few significant effects. One was that case management increased the possibility of higher utilization of formal support services, and the other was that psychotherapy for caregivers delayed institutionalization for the patients. We already noted that computer networking had a positive effect on the decision-making skills of the caregivers. However, this last intervention was also found wanting on several other outcome measures. Overall, the findings of this review were discouraging. The authors described many serious methodological shortcoming that might have impacted on the outcome.

One randomized controlled trial investigated the outcome of social networking for the caregivers of persons with dementia (Charlesworth, Tzimoula, Higgs, and Poland, 2007). They tested the following hypotheses: (1) Regular support from family and friends would be most available for caregivers with family-dependent and locally integrated network types, which were separated into five categories – family dependent, locally integrated, local self-contained, wider community-focused, and private-restricted; (2) admission into permanent residential/nursing care would be less common for caregivers with locally integrated, family-dependent networks; and (3) the befriending intervention would most likely be used by those caregivers with locally self-contained and private-restricted support networks.

A total of 236 caregivers were randomly assigned into a Befriending and Cost of Caring (BECCA) trial. The results showed that the mean age of the caregivers was 68 years and the mean age of the person with dementia was 78 years. Most of the participants (80%) were living with the person with dementia. Half of all the caregivers received some form of daily support from family, friends, or neighbours, but under one-third received no such support. Caregivers in the family-dependent and locally-integrated networks received regular support. Caregivers in the broader community-focused networks received only occasional support. The majority of caregivers were in the private-restricted network and had no or only limited family or friends and received very little support. The results showed that caregivers in the locally integrated and local self-contained categories were most likely to have their relatives institutionalized. However, the most critical finding of this study was that the type of support system at the baseline was only marginally significant in relation to the institutionalization of the person with dementia.

This unique study investigated the predictive power of network typology, and what was found was that the patterns of family support, use of befriending, and institutionalization of the person with dementia varied with the caregiver network typology. The authors concluded by acknowledging that policy and practice had to include assessments of the caregiver's network as an integral part of an assessment to determine and develop a network of support systems to provide respite.

Charlesworth, Shepstone, and associates (2008), in a further analysis of the data reported above, concluded that there was no evidence for a benefit of access to a 'befriender' facilitator on outcomes which were improving psychological well-being and quality of life for caregivers of persons with dementia.

Thompson and colleagues (2007) conducted a systematic review of 44 studies that broadly included three types of interventions: (1)

technology-based (4 studies); (2) group-based (13 studies) and (3) individual-based (27 studies). The results of these interventions, on the whole, were disappointing. Only group interventions (with psycho-educational foundations) had a positive impact on depression in the caregivers. The clinical value of these improvements was uncertain. A major problem encountered in this kind of review is the sheer hetero-geneity of outcome measures. For example, providing information and support alone is rare in the interventions of caregivers of persons with dementia. The authors noted that what may be termed support often incorporated broader interventions such as problem-solving, psycho-educational training, and so on. The main conclusion of this review was that there existed little evidence that interventions designed to support and provide information to caregivers of persons with dementia were uniformly effective.

Our final review of the value of technologies supporting caregivers of people with dementia (Powell, Chiu, & Eysenbach, 2008) was not any more encouraging than the preceding reviews. Out of a total of 1456 abstracts reviewed, only 15 papers describing five interventions were included in this review. The outcome measure included the caregiv-er's health status, quality of life, burden, and satisfaction, the service utilization, and costs. The outcomes were inconsistent, but there was some evidence that some information-based technology interventions might have had some moderating effect on improving caregiver stress and depression. The treatment effects were influenced by factors such as ethnicity, formal support, and baseline-burden. The authors con-cluded that, theoretically, information-based technology interventions have the potential of alleviating the burden of caring and prolonging community living for the persons with dementia. Further research was called for to fully assess the true value of information-based technology interventions.

Summary

The benefits of social support interventions for caregivers are far from self-evident. There exists an array of interventions ranging from pro-fessional type groups and individual therapeutic interventions to information-based technology and support programs to enhance the support circle for the caregiver. Outcome measures were also varied. Very few statistically significant outcomes were reported. The clinical significance of some of the interventions was equally in doubt. This picture is discouraging, as the burden of caring on the health and well-being of caregivers of persons with dementia is considerable.

Conclusion

The term 'social support interventions' is problematic. A narrow definition would imply only those types of interventions specifically designed to promote social support for the caregivers of persons with dementia. Our search, however, yielded a wide range of interventions encompassing individual psychotherapy and technology-based interventions. Peer support groups or volunteer-based programs which may be representative of social support interventions that would enhance the support system for the caregiver were not well represented in our review.

This chapter was divided into three parts, dealing with, first, a mix of studies ranging from smoking cessation to prolongation of longevity by church attenders; second, breast cancer; and third, dementia. Our aim was to assess the benefits of social support interventions with these conditions. With the group of mixed studies, the findings were somewhat ambiguous. Review of the outcome studies of social support interventions yielded mixed and unconvincing outcomes. Many of the studies seemed to be promising, but failed to reach statistically significant results.

The result of our foray into the breast cancer literature was encouraging. While the social support interventions showed promise, any generalized conclusion was not possible due to the extraordinary array of outcome measures these studies adopted. Yet, the major reviews on the effectiveness of social support interventions with persons with breast cancer were promising.

Finally, the outcome of social support literature with persons with dementia and their caregivers suffered from some of the same problems noted above. The effectiveness of these interventions were less than promising. Unfortunately, one central problem, the high level of morbidity in the caregivers of persons with dementia, remained unaddressed. Depression in the caregiver and delaying institutionalization of the dementia patient were two measures commonly reported. Again, the results were promising without being statistically significant. A problem noted above, that is, what constitutes social support intervention, remained unclear in the studies reported here.

In sum, the effectiveness of social support interventions remains questionable. First, a much tighter definition for interventions in this category is called for. Second, one of the key outcome measures must be related to reducing the burden factor in the caregivers, thereby eliminating or minimizing their risk for morbidity. In the meantime, common sense and clinical observations dictate that social support intervention (of any kind) with the caregiver is better than no intervention.

REFERENCES

Charlesworth, G., Shepstone, L., Wilson, E., Reynolds, S., et al. (2008). Befriending carers of people with dementia: Randomized controlled trial. *BMJ, 336*, 1295–1297.

Charlesworth, G., Tzimoula, X., Higgs, P., & Poland, F. (2007). Social networks, befriending and support for family carers of people with dementia. *Quality in Aging – Policy, Practice and Research, 8*, 37–44.

Edwards, A., Hulbert-Williams, N., & Neal, N. (2008). Psychological interventions for women with metastatic breast cancer. *Cochrane Database Systematic Review, Issue 3*, art. no.: DOI: 10.1002/14651858.CD004253.pub3.

Krause, N. (2006). Church-based social support and mortality. *J. Gerontology, 61B*, s140–s146.

May, S , & West, R. (2000). Do social support interventions (buddy systems) aid smoking cessation? A review. *Tobacco Control, 9*: 415–422.

May, S., West, R., Hajek, P., McEwen, A., & McRobbie, H. (2006). Randomized controlled trial of a social support (buddy) intervention for smoking cessation. *Patient Education and Counseling, 64*, 235–241.

Napoles-Springer, A., Ortiz, C., O'Brien, H., & Diaz-Mendez, M. (2009). Developing a culturally competent peer support intervention for Spanish speaking Latinas with breast cancer. *J. Immigrant Minority Health, 11*, 268–280.

Nausheen, B., Gidron, Y., Peveler, R., & Moss-Morris, R. (2009). Social support and cancer progression: A systematic review. *J. Psychosomatic Research, 67*, 403–415.

O'Connor, D., Ames, D., Gardner, B., & King, M. (2009). Psychosocial treatments of psychological symptoms in dementia: A systematic review of reports meeting quality standards. *International Psychogeriatrics, 21*, 241–251.

Peacock, S. & Forbes, D. (2003). Interventions for caregivers of persons with dementia: A systematic review. *Canadian J. Nursing Research, 35*, 88–107.

Pistrang, N., Barker, C., & Humphreys, K. (2008). Mutual help groups for mental health problems: A review of effective studies. *Am. J. Community Psychology, 42*, 110–121.

Powell, J., Chiu, T., & Eysenbach, G. (2008). A systematic review of network technologies supporting carers of people with dementia. *J. Telemedicine and Telecare, 14*, 154–156.

Salonen, P., Tarkka, M., Kellokumpu-Lehtinen, P., Astedt-Kurki, P., Luukkaala, T., et al. (2009). Telephone intervention and quality of life in patients with breast cancer. *Cancer Nursing, 32*, 177–190.

Spijker, A., Vernooij-Dassen, M., Vasse, E., Adang, E., et al. (2008). Effectiveness of non-pharmacological interventions in delaying the institutionalization of patients with dementia: A Meta-Analysis. *J. Am. Geriatric Soc., 56*, 1116–1128.

Thompson, C., Spilsbury, K., Hall, J., Birks, Y., et al. (2007). Systemic review of information and support interventions for caregivers of people with dementia. *BMC Geriatrics, 7*, 18–35.

van Dam, H., van der Horst, F., Knoops, L., Ryckman, R., et. al. (2005). Social support in diabetes: A systematic review of controlled intervention studies. *Patient Education and Counseling, 59*, 1–12.

Watt, R., Tull, K., Hardy, R., Wiggins, M., et al. (2008). Effectiveness of a social support intervention on infant feeding practices: Randomized control trial. *J. Epidemiology and Community Health, 63*, 156–162.

10 Afterthoughts

At the time of writing this book a story broke involving the death of an old man in a fire. Sad, but not an unusual story in itself. But it was unusual for the simple fact that the firefighters could not get inside the house to rescue the man due to the sheer volume of clutter blocking the front door and hallway. Neighbours were concerned about their isolated neighbour, but they did not want to invade his privacy. This is a sad story for many reasons. From our point of view, however, his death was caused by profound social isolation. At the other end of this sad saga, I have a friend who has been involved with young mothers with small children (who often experience social isolation), coming together with them once a week for prayers and conversations at their church. These two stories tell us that social isolation is endemic to modern urban living, and yet all kinds of wonderful activities go on in our community every day to counter this problem and promote social support.

The state of the family in much of the Western world is one of turmoil. The nuclear family is in rapid decline and divorce is ubiquitous. Single-mother families, also the poorest in our society, abound. More and more people, by choice, live alone. Social institutions such as church and clubs play a smaller and smaller role in our lives. Under these circumstances, the availability of intimates may not be taken for granted. Yet, exactly what might supplant intimate support remains obscure. Social isolation in urban centres abounds. Many social organizations have attempted to fill this gap.

In doing research for this book, a number of questions came to my mind, such as who provides support (we know that spousal/partner support is very effective), how often and how much, and with what consequences. Family and friends are often the most common sources of support. Unfortunately, they may not always be available. Does this suggest a deliberate effort driven by policy to ensure that support is made available to the more vulnerable members of our society? Still, there are innumerable support groups in the community offering a whole range of services – from meals on wheels for the housebound to peer support groups (Compassionate Friends) for parents who experience the death of a child. In Winnipeg, Manitoba, a community-based program for the elderly, Age and Opportunity, offers a variety of programs ranging from exercise classes to weekly luncheons to foreign holidays. By definition, people who participate in the activities of Age and Opportunity are relatively well. It is a different story for the housebound, chronically ill person. If we agree that social support promotes health (and in the case of the elderly safety is often a major concern), then the need for comprehensive social support programs that include regular home visits is imperative. On the other hand, we cannot confirm with any degree of confidence the buffering effects of these types of community support. Prima facie, they may not represent a true alternative to intimate support.

The multidimensional nature of social support was somewhat of a revelation. The buffering function of social support is generally supported in the literature. Spousal support generally predicts a positive outcome in dealing with an illness, but not necessarily. The main effect or the buffering function is most powerful when the partner relationship is characterized by reciprocity. There is the right but also the wrong kind of social support. Sources of social support are so wide ranging as to defy any simple categorization. Yet, effective social support has the capacity to have a positive influence on the course and outcome of illness.

The title of this book suggests that the relationship between social support and health is complicated. This was borne out in many different ways. In relation to clinical depression (chapter 5), we noted that while spousal/partner support was a positive force, there was also a darker side. Conflictual marriages predicted serious problems, especially for women with this affliction. Breast cancer (chapter 7) can have very positive effects on conflictual marital relationships. Long-standing marriage relationships appear to be very beneficial for breast cancer patients. On the other hand, caregivers (especially spouses) of persons with dementia (chapter 6) are vulnerable to developing physical and psychological problems. The burden of caregiving is very pronounced in these caregivers. HIV/AIDS sufferers (chapter 8) rely on each other for support more so any other group we examined in this book. Spouses of chronic pain sufferers (chapter 4) may overprotect their partners, thus perpetuating pain behaviours. Social support is a good thing, but it is truly not that simple.

One objective in my writing this book is to alert the clinical community to the fact that social support has a central place in the overall assessment of a patient. Whether a patient is being discharged to home after surgery, or a child is diagnosed with a serious medical condition, social support may have a significant impact on how these situations are handled. The research leaves little doubt about the preventive and curative power of intimate social support. We also learned that not all social support is positive. In simple terms, too much kindness and over-involvement may be counter-productive. Each case has to be judged against the reality and specifics of a given situation. To date, it can be stated with some confidence that social support, in all its complexity, has not made its way into the routine assessment of patients. The cost of this oversight cannot be easily estimated.

Finally, we need to reiterate that research into the thorny question of the main effects versus buffering hypothesis is not yet fully resolved. Perhaps these phenomena coexist, and at times which is more dominant is difficult to sort out. An incontrovertible truth is that marriage or being in an intimate relationship (as opposed to being single) does reduce morbidity and prolong life. A second point is that our focus has clearly been on the power of intimate social support, focusing where we could on marital/partner relationships. We adopted this approach for the simple reason that the buffering effect of spousal support appears to be predominant. Yet, we can conceive of many situations where such support is not tenable. We noted that the family structure in the West has undergone a virtual revolution, with sharp increases in one-person and single-mother households. Intimate social support is often not a viable option for these individuals, and thoughts must be given to organized programs that would broadly counteract some of the profoundly negative consequences of single parenthood or living alone.

Author Index

Subject Index

Age and Opportunity (support group), 172
AIDS. *See* HIV/AIDS
Alzheimer's disease, ix, x, 101–2, 104, 106, 107, 110, 113. *See also* dementia
arthritis, 44, 66; Juvenile Chronic Arthritis, 26, 28, 31, 32
asthma. *See under* childhood illnesses

back pain. *See* chronic low-back pain
'Bio–Dad' (television program), 47
breast cancer, 119–37; and body image, 121, 122–3, 129, 135, 136, 137; and buffering hypothesis of social support, 121, 131–7; caregiver burden, 120; communication patterns between patients and their partners (study), 127–8; and depression, 120, 123, 133–5, 136, 137; depression in partners of breast cancer patients, 128, 130; diagnosis of, 120, 121; and effectiveness of social support interventions, 128, 131–7, 156, 160–3, 168; and emotional distress, 120–3; factors that brought patients and their partners closer (study), 130–1; impact of marital satisfaction on women who had a mastectomy (study), 135–6; influence of psychosocial factors on (study), 131; influence of social network on cancer mortality (study), 131–2; mutuality of distress in cancer patients and their partners, 123–4, 131; partner adaptation to, 124–5; partner-related issues, 123–31, 137; power of marriage to prolong life for cancer patients, 132–3, 137; physical symptoms of, 122; problems experienced by patients and their partners (study), 125; reactions and adjustment of partners, 128–31; role of social support in the early stages of, 133–4; and stress-buffering effect of personal control, 120–1; value of partner support, 43–4, 136, 172; in young women, 122–3. *See also* cancer
buffering effect of social support, ix–x, 4, 5, 8–22, 45, 172; buffering effect of intimate relationships,